Making WISE CHOICES

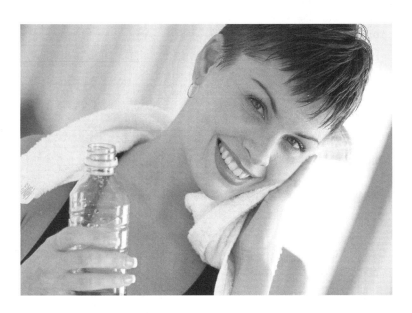

Gospel Light

FIRST PLACE™

Gospel Light is a Christian publisher dedicated to serving the local church. We believe God's vision for Gospel Light is to provide church leaders with biblical, user-friendly materials that will help them evangelize, disciple and minister to children, youth and families.

It is our prayer that this Gospel Light resource will help you discover biblical truth for your own life and help you minister to others. May God richly bless you.

For a free catalog of resources from Gospel Light, please contact your Christian supplier or contact us at 1-800-4-GOSPEL or www.gospellight.com.

PUBLISHING STAFF
William T. Greig, Chairman
Kyle Duncan, Publisher
Dr. Elmer L. Towns, Senior Consulting Publisher
Pam Weston, Senior Editor
Patti Pennington Virtue, Associate Editor
Kathryn T. Schuh, Editorial Assistant
Hilary Young, Editorial Assistant
Bayard Taylor, M.Div., Senior Editor, Biblical and Theological Issues
Samantha A. Hsu, Cover Production and Internal Designer
June Chapko, Contributing Writer

ISBN 0-8307-3081-8
© 2002 First Place
All rights reserved.
Printed in the U.S.A.

Any omission of credits is unintentional. The publisher requests documentation for future printings.

CAUTION
The information contained in this book is intended to be solely informational and educational. It is assumed that the First Place participant will consult a medical or health professional before beginning this or any other weight-loss or physical-fitness program.

CONTENTS

FOREWORD

My introduction to Bible study came when I joined First Place in March of 1981. I had been in church since I was a small child, but the extent of my study of the Bible had been reading my Sunday School quarterly on Saturday night. On Sunday morning, I would listen to my Sunday School teacher as she taught God's Word to me. During the worship service, I would listen to our pastor as he taught God's Word to me. Digging out the truths of the Bible for myself had frankly never entered my mind.

Perhaps you are right where I was back in 1981. If so, you are in for a blessing you never dreamed possible. As you start studying the truths of the Bible for yourself, you will see God begin to open your understanding of His Word. Bible study is one of the nine commitments of the First Place program. The First Place Bible studies are designed to be done on a daily basis. Each day's study will take approximately 15 to 20 minutes to complete, but you will be discovering the deep truths of God's Word as you work through each week's study.

There are many in-depth Bible studies on the market. The First Place Bible studies are not designed for the purpose of in-depth study. They are designed to be used in conjunction with the other eight commitments of the program to bring balance into our lives. Our desire is for each member to begin having a personal quiet time with God each day. This time alone with God should include a time of prayer, Bible reading and Bible study. Having a quiet time is a daily discipline that will bring the rich rewards of balance, something we all need.

A part of each week's study is the Bible memory verse for the week. You will find a CD at the back of this Bible study that contains all 10 of the memory verses for the study set to music. The CD has an upbeat tempo suitable for use when exercising. The songs help you to memorize the verses easily and retain them for future reference. If you memorize Scripture as you study, God will use His Word to transform your life.

Almost every First Place member I have talked with about the program says, "The weight loss is wonderful, but the most important thing I have received from my association with First Place is learning to study God's Word."

God bless you as you begin this exciting journey toward a balanced life. God will richly bless your efforts to give Him first place in your life. Remember Matthew 6:33: "But seek first his kingdom and his righteousness, and all these things will be given to you as well."

Carole Lewis
First Place National Director

INTRODUCTION

The First Place Bible studies were developed to be used in conjunction with the First Place weight-loss program. However, the studies could also be used by anyone who desires to learn more about God's Word and His will, with the added bonus of learning more about living a healthy lifestyle.

A Balanced Life

First Place is a Christ-centered health program, emphasizing balance in the physical, mental, emotional and spiritual areas of life. The First Place program is meant to be a daily process. As we learn to keep Christ first in our lives, we will find that He is the One who satisfies our hunger and our every need.

God's Word contains guidelines for maintaining our physical well-being, equipping us mentally to make right choices, providing emotional stability to handle everyday circumstances as well as crisis situations, and growing spiritually as we deepen our relationship with Him.

The Nine Commitments

The First Place program has nine commitments that will help you draw closer to the Lord and aid you in establishing a solid, consistent and healthy Christian life. Each commitment is a necessary and important part of the goal of First Place to help you become healthier and stronger in all areas of your life—living the abundant life He has planned for each of us. To help you achieve growth in all four areas, First Place asks you to keep these nine commitments:

1. Attendance
2. Encouragement
3. Prayer
4. Bible reading
5. Scripture memory verse
6. Bible study
7. Live-It plan
8. Commitment Record
9. Exercise

The Components

There are six distinct components to this Bible study to aid you in bringing balance to your life. These components include the 10-week Bible study, 6 Wellness Worksheets, 2 weeks of menu plans, the leader's discussion guide, 13 Commitment Records and the Scripture Memory Music CD.

The Bible Study

Each week of each 10-week Bible study is divided into five daily assignments with Days 6 and 7 set aside for reflections on the week's lesson. The following guidelines will help make your study more enjoyable and profitable:

- Set aside 15 to 20 minutes each day to complete the daily assignment. It's best not to attempt to complete a week's worth of Bible study in one day.
- Pray before each day's study and ask God to give you understanding and a teachable heart.
- Keep in mind that the ultimate goal of Bible study is not for knowledge only but also for application and a changed life.
- First Place suggests using the *New International Version* of the Bible to complete the studies.
- Don't feel anxious if you can't seem to find the *correct* answer. Many times the Word will speak differently to different people, depending upon where they are in their walk with God and the season of life they are experiencing.
- Be prepared to discuss with your fellow First Place members what you learned that week through your study.

Wellness Worksheets

The informative and interactive Wellness Worksheets have been developed by Dr. Jody Wilkinson of the Cooper Institute in Dallas, Texas. These worksheets are intended to help you understand and achieve balance in all four areas of your life: physical, mental, emotional and spiritual. Your leader will assign specific worksheets as At-Home Assignments throughout the 13-week session.

Menu Plans

The two-week menu plans were developed especially for First Place by Chef Scott Wilson. Each menu is meant to simplify meal planning and include food exchanges. These meals are based on the MasterCook software that uses a database of over 6,000 food items, which was prepared using United States Department of Agriculture (USDA) publications and information from food manufacturers.

Leader's Discussion Guide

This discussion guide is provided to help the First Place leader guide a group through this Bible study. It provides information for the leader to prepare for each weekly group meeting.

Personal Weight Record

The Personal Weight Record is for the member to use to keep a record of weight loss. After the weigh-in at each week's meeting, the member will record any loss or gain on the chart.

Commitment Records

Thirteen Commitment Records (CRs) are provided in the back of this Bible study. For your convenience these have been printed on perforated paper so that you may easily remove them from the book and carry them with you through each week as you keep your First Place commitments. Directions for filling out the CRs precedes those pages.

Scripture Memory CD

Since Scripture memory music is such a vital part of the First Place program, the Scripture Memory Music CD for this study is included in the back inside cover. The verses for this study are set to music that can be listened to as you work, play or travel. The CD can be an effective tool as you exercise since the first verse is set to music with a warm-up tempo, the next eight verses are set to workout tempo, and the music of the last verse can be used for a cooldown.

GOD'S COMMAND

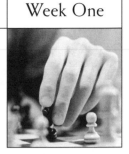

MEMORY VERSE

This day I call heaven and earth as witnesses against you that I have set before you life and death, blessings and curses. Now choose life, so that you and your children may live.

Deuteronomy 30:19

Each day we make a myriad of choices, from the seemingly mundane—whether to wear the blue jacket or the beige one—to the life altering—which job offer to accept—and everything in between. In choosing to join First Place, you have begun a journey to exciting choices yet to be made.

Serious decisions require serious thought. In this week's study, you will learn how important it is to make the right choices, how to discern wisely and the consequences for wrong choices.

DAY 1: *Life and Death*

All day long we make choices; some that are not so important and others that affect our lives and the lives of others. God has given us the freedom to choose.

➢ According to Deuteronomy 30:19, what are the choices we are offered by God?

When we choose life, we receive blessings from God. "Blessings" is a wonderful term used in the Bible to describe many things, including salvation, having a relationship with God, experiencing peace and enjoying life.

≫ As you choose to eat healthy and honor the commitments you have made to God through First Place, what are some of the blessings you might receive?

A closer relationship with God, more energy, a positive outlook, longer life and a healthier body are but a few of the possible blessings that come from choosing to honor your nine First Place commitments.

If we choose death, we receive curses. The word "curses" translated in the original text means the opposite of blessings.

≫ Name some possible consequences of making unhealthy choices.

Depression, diseases, weight gain, high blood pressure, shorter life span and a mediocre relationship with the Lord are common to those who regularly make unwise lifestyle choices.

When you joined First Place, you made a commitment to God and asked Him to help you live a healthier lifestyle. He has set before you the choice between life and blessings or death and curses.

≫ Which will you choose?   ☐ Life   ☐ Death

Write a prayer in your journal thanking God for the opportunity to make wise choices and for the blessings He offers when we choose life. Continue to prayerfully ask Him to guide you over the coming weeks as you seek to choose foods and establish habits which will restore your body to good health.

Heavenly Father, I am so thankful that You have provided me with the ability to choose between life and death.

Lord, I choose life. Thank You for the blessings You have promised in Your Word. Fill me with Your wisdom, that I might choose what is Your perfect will in every aspect of my life.

DAY 2: *Blessings in Obedience*

We all make at least some wise choices in different areas of our lives. Have you ever chosen to stop at a yellow light even though you were in a hurry—only to discover when the light turned green that a policeman was parked just around the corner waiting to catch someone going through a red light? Your wise choice to be a minute or two late in getting to your destination probably saved you a much longer delay if you had sped through the light and then been caught and ticketed by the officer.

Think about choices you have made over the past several months. Were there situations in which you could have made negative choices but opted for positive ones? There are so many areas to consider, including physical, financial, relational and spiritual.

➤ List three positive choices you have recently made; then list the negative choices you could have made. (These could include physical, financial, relational and spiritual choices.)

Positive Choices	Negative Choices

➤ In what ways did you benefit from making the wiser choices?

According to Deuteronomy 28:1-2, when we obey the Lord and follow His commands, we receive His blessings.

> ⁕ What are some areas of your life in which you have not been obedient to God's commands?

> ⁕ What are some of the blessings that are listed in Deuteronomy 28:3-13 and how do these blessings relate to modern day life (i.e., many of us do not have livestock or crops, but we do have our jobs; how does this blessing relate to our jobs)?

Ask God to help you obey His commands and show you the blessings He has for you.

 Dear God, please help me be obedient and do the things You want me to do. I want to be consistent, Lord, in all that I do, so You will be glorified. You know my sins, my shortcomings and my weaknesses; please help me especially in these areas, guiding me and helping me to overcome them.

DAY 3: *Enemies Defeated*

According to Deuteronomy 28:7, the enemies were those who would rise up against those who obeyed God's commands. Have you ever made a decision to do something you know God wants you to do only to have obstacles block your way and enemies rise up to thwart your success?

> ⁕ Name some enemies you might encounter as you begin to live a healthier lifestyle.

➤ Making a change in your lifestyle for the better tends to bring out well-meaning critics. Which of the following statements have you heard? (Check all that apply.)

☐ Don't lose too much weight; you'll get sick.

☐ Everyone in our family has a large frame; you're not fat.

☐ You should try that famous star diet; she dropped 20 pounds in the first week.

☐ Just use willpower and the pounds will melt away.

If you are a child of God and trying to obey Him, you can expect Satan's opposition. His name means "adversary" and "accuser." Satan will tempt you and try to destroy the things in your life that will bring glory to God.

➤ In Deuteronomy 28:7, what does God promise will happen to your enemies?

They will come at you from _____ direction, but _____ from you in _____.

God will pulverize your enemies one by one, sending them scattering in seven different directions. Just as nocturnal animals scatter in bright light, so your enemies will be eliminated when the light of the Holy Spirit exposes them.

According to Deuteronomy 1:29-30, God does not want you to live in fear. He goes before you and fights for you. If you pay attention, you will see the results of God's army fighting for you in the victories that are won.

➤ What do you consider to be the biggest enemy you face today?

Have you talked to God about the enemies in your life? Your journal is a wonderful way to record your fears and God's reassuring answers. Go to Him now—ask Him to scatter your enemies and thank Him for the victory.

Father God, calm my fears and drive out the enemies that would cause me to stumble. Please go before me—clearing the way and giving me the wisdom I need to change my eating habits for a healthy lifestyle. I will give You all the glory for the victory.

DAY 4: *Certain Victory*

Wouldn't it be grand to have success guaranteed? To know that no matter what we attempted to accomplish in our career, home, finances, church, hobbies, etc., they would all turn into victory?

➻ If you could do anything and know you would succeed, what would you want to do?

➻ What prevents you from taking the first step toward achieving what you want to do? What obstacles are in your way?

As you move toward your goals in First Place, allowing God to guide you and disperse your enemies, you will experience one small victory after another.

➻ What does God promise in Deuteronomy 28:8?

The Lord will send a blessing on your barns and on _____ you put your _____ to.

➻ What area in your life do you feel is most in need of God's blessing?

➤ Are you ready to trust God by putting this area of your life into His hands?

☐ Yes   ☐ No

➤ Why or why not?

Pray the following prayer of obedience. Write your prayer and your goals in your prayer journal, asking God to take the need in your life and the goals of your heart and bring them together in victory.

Precious Lord, my heart's desire is to be obedient to You. I am willing to listen and obey whatever You want me to do. I fail so many times, but I know that as I confess my disobedience, You are gracious to forgive me. Help me now, Lord, as I commit to following You and doing Your will. I depend on You, trusting You because You love me and want only good in my life.

DAY 5: *God's Holy People*

An oath is a sacred promise and something to be valued highly. A marriage vow and an oath of office are two examples of commitments that we do not take lightly.

The oath God gives in Deuteronomy 28:9 has two parts: His part and your part.

➤ What is God's promise?

The word "establish" means "to bring into existence; to make firm or stable; to introduce and cause to grow and multiply; to set up."[1] God has done what He has promised—brought His holy people into existence, set them up firmly and caused them to grow and multiply.

≫ What is your part in this promise?

≫ Read the following verses and write the key thought of each concerning oaths:

• Numbers 30:1-2

• Deuteronomy 23:21

• Psalm 116:12-14

• Ecclesiastes 5:2-7

≫ Reread Deuteronomy 28:1-14. You have a choice—to obey God or not. Which will you choose?

God loves you just the way you are, no matter what you choose. He gives each of us the opportunity to make wise choices. We have been given a free will and we can choose to go our own way, doing whatever pleases us in the moment, or we can choose to freely love God and do what He wants, taking a long-term view of reality.

≫ How will you pray, telling God you will do your part, so that He may do His part? Write your prayer here or in your prayer journal.

DAY 6: *Reflections*

This week you have learned the importance of obedience to God. From the very beginning in the Garden of Eden, obedience has been a matter of choice. When you choose to obey God, you will experience blessings beyond understanding.

God designed blessings to be the outcome of obedience. When you trust Him and choose to do what He commands, you will experience the immediate blessing of pleasing God. In John 8:29, Jesus said, "I always do what pleases him." Pleasing God means obeying Him. Jesus' goal was to please His Father, even unto death.

You, too, can demonstrate your goal of pleasing God by your obedience to Him. In the First Place program, there are nine commitments to fulfill between you and God. Fulfilling each of these every day will please God, and you will experience His wonderful blessings week after week as you move toward your healthy lifestyle goals.

God waits for you to call upon Him for help when you stumble upon a rough spot in the road. He wants to reach out to you and pull you up. Obedience to God is a partnership where you do your part and God does His. Knowing that can make your First Place journey less intimidating and more doable.

 Father God, thank You for the opportunity through faith in Christ and the power of the Holy Spirit to choose to be obedient. My commitment to You is made because You have loved me first—and, as a result, I trust and love You. My obedience is evidence of that love (see John 14:21).

Lord, thank You for all the blessings You have given me as a result of choosing to be obedient to You (see 1 John 3:22).

Father in heaven, I want my goal to always be to please You. Help me to be obedient in all things. I know You will always fulfill your part and I commit to doing mine (see 2 Corinthians 5:9).

DAY 7: *Reflections*

Obedience is not always easy. Satan does not want God's people doing what pleases God. While Satan knows he cannot have the Christian's soul, he will attempt to destroy our testimonies by enticing us into making bad choices.

Like a roaring lion, Satan goes about looking for someone facing difficult situations or disheartened by life's challenges (see 1 Peter 5:8). He offers us the choice of temporary escape from hard times through deceit and cunning ways.

God will never abandon you. He will disperse your enemies before your eyes, bringing you through the difficult times to victory. Compare your enemy to a walnut being smashed and the pieces flying in all directions. That will give you an idea of God's wrath upon those who would dare try to bring you down.

Each time you choose to obey God and experience His blessing, you become stronger. Victory upon victory will strengthen you, better equipping you to stand firm in the face of temptation. Remember: Temptation does not come from God (see James 1:13-14). C. S. Lewis once said that suffering is what God brings into our lives to knock us off our self-centeredness and to become more loving. Obedience will build our spiritual muscles and strengthen us to withstand the temptations of the devil with the goal of producing godly love in our lives.

Thank You, God, for being there with me during times of danger and temptations. Your presence assures me I am not destined to fail but to emerge victorious, giving You the glory (see Joshua 1:5).

Father, I am grateful that what I choose to do in obedience to You is not in vain. Help me to always stand firm and give myself fully to Your work (see 1 Corinthians 15:58).

Lord, help me resist the devil's tricks. My desire is to be self-controlled and alert. Thank You for standing with me and helping me to emerge victorious (see 1 Peter 5:8).

Note
1. *Merriam-Webster's Collegiate Dictionary*, 10th ed., s.v. "establish."

GROUP PRAYER REQUESTS   TODAY'S DATE:_____

NAME	REQUEST	RESULTS

THE BALANCED LIFE

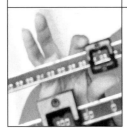

MEMORY VERSE
Jesus grew in wisdom and stature,
and in favor with God and men.
Luke 2:52

The First Place logo contains the four aspects mentioned in this week's memory verse: wisdom (mental), stature (physical), in favor with God (spiritual), and in favor with men (emotional).

In Matthew 6:33, Jesus said, "Seek first his kingdom and his righteousness, and all these things will be given to you as well." When you place Jesus first in your life, your life will be well balanced. In this week's study, we will examine each of these four aspects of our lives. Every day you are faced with choices that may affect the balance of your life. Let's learn how to make wise choices in every area of life.

DAY 1: *Mental Growth*

According to Luke 2:41-47, at the age of 12 Jesus spent several days among the teachers in the Temple courts in Jerusalem.

> After three days [Mary and Joseph] found him in the temple courts, sitting among the teachers, listening to them and asking them questions. Everyone who heard him was amazed at his understanding and his answers (vv. 46-47).

Notice that Jesus was *listening* to the teachers. Have you ever been so busy talking that you didn't really listen to what was being said? When someone is speaking to you, are you mentally preparing your answer while that person is speaking, instead of really listening to what's being said? Perhaps you get distracted thinking about other events or concerns in your life. God wants you to listen and give your full attention to Him, not only as you read Scripture, but also when you pray, hear a sermon or listen to an inspirational message.

➤ What does James 1:19 say about the importance of listening?

➤ According to John 10:27, why is it important to recognize our Shepherd's voice?

Jesus was also *asking questions*. How often have you asked questions in your First Place class? Asking questions can supply answers, not only for yourself, but also for others. Taking notes while listening to sermons or speakers is a great way to formulate questions while gaining an understanding of what you are hearing.

➤ What is the promise found in Jeremiah 33:3?

➤ Although most would interpret Matthew 7:7-8 to be a teaching on prayer, how does it relate to the topic of mental growth?

Do you have a *teachable spirit*? If a person is not willing to be taught, it's difficult for him or her to gain understanding. Mental growth requires effort and a desire to learn. If we are willing to take the time and expend the energy required, we will be rewarded with increased understanding.

➤ Read Proverbs 1:7. Do you have a teachable spirit that does not "despise wisdom and discipline"? How do you react when someone tries to teach or correct you?

Listening, asking questions and having a teachable spirit will lead you to *understanding*. Can you recall a time when you suddenly realized that you really understood something you had been trying to grasp? The people in the Temple courts were amazed at Jesus' answers that showed that He understood—and remember, He was only 12 years old!

➤ According to Proverbs 2:1-12, what are the benefits of gaining understanding?

➤ Of the four steps to mental growth—listening, asking questions, being teachable and gaining understanding—which is easiest for you? Which of these steps is an area that you need to work on?

When we take time to listen and to ask questions, and we desire to be taught, we will gain understanding. Each day we are faced with many choices on how to spend our time. Spend some of your precious time each day in learning new things. Reading and memorizing Scripture, reading a book that challenges you to think or listening to a good teacher are all worthwhile pursuits.

 Heavenly Father, thank You that You have promised to answer when I call to You and to teach me great and unsearchable things (see Jeremiah 33:3). Help me, Lord, to have a teachable spirit and to listen to You for the answers I need.

DAY 2: *Physical Development*

Luke 2:52 tells us that not only did Jesus grow in wisdom, but also in stature. The definition of "stature" is "quality or status gained by growth, development or achievement."[1]

From what we know about Jesus' adult life, we can surmise that He was physically fit. We know that He walked considerably, and we know that many of the roads He traveled were rough and uneven. We also know He was a carpenter by trade—a strenuous occupation. He even managed to walk up the hill to His crucifixion after having been beaten by the guards after His arrest. This could not have been accomplished if Jesus had not maintained a healthy body.

➢ Think back to when you were about 12 years old. What was your physical stature like (i.e., were you tall and thin, short and stocky, petite, fragile, etc.)?

➢ Check any activities in which you were involved while growing up.

☐ Bike riding	☐ Running
☐ Skating (any type)	☐ Climbing
☐ Swimming	☐ Hiking
☐ Team sports	☐ Dance/gymnastics
☐ Other _____	

➢ How did you feel when participating in these activities?

➢ Which do you still participate in?

≫ What are the benefits of being physically active?

≫ If being physically active is an area that you need to work on, what is one thing that you can do this week to add more physical activity in your life? (**Note:** If you are not now doing regular physical activity, please consult your regular physician before beginning any vigorous activity.)

Parents are always concerned about the development and physical growth of their children. We want our children to be healthy and strong, and God, our heavenly Father, wants nothing less for us. When we are physically strong, we are better able to withstand the rigors of daily life and to serve Him.

 Precious Lord, I want to be all that You desire for me. There are times when I feel helpless and don't want to get up and get moving. Give me Your strength and power to begin again. I want to be fit and healthy to serve You. Show me what I can do this week to strengthen my body.

DAY 3: *Spiritual Maturity*

The Greek word for "favor," used in Luke 2:52, is *charis*, which means divine influence upon the heart and the reflection of that influence in one's life. It also means gift, grace, joy, pleasure and gratitude.

≫ Read James 1:4 and fill in the blanks.

Perseverance must finish its work so that you may be

_____ and _____,

not lacking anything.

A sign of spiritual maturity is making choices that are pleasing to God. God wants our lives to be a reflection of His love for us. A spiritually mature person can be used by God to show Himself to others. As you mature spiritually, the door will be opened for you to share the hope that is in Christ. Even your imperfections can be used by God to show that His love doesn't depend on our perfection, but on *His*. Only as we grow in our relationship with God can we be perfected according to His will.

> Four of the nine First Place commitments are spiritually based; name them.

It pleases God when you choose to have a quiet prayer time, reading and studying His Word and memorizing Scripture verses. In doing these things you continue to grow spiritually. You are growing in favor with God by allowing His divine influence upon your heart to be reflected in your life.

> With which of the four spiritual First Place commitments do you need help?

> What will you do this week to work on that particular commitment?

Babies are adorable, and it is fun to watch them grow and learn new things. What would happen if a child grew to adult size but refused to grow up emotionally? When people become Christians, they are spiritual babies. Unfortunately, there are many Christians who never get past their infant stage spiritually. If we do nothing to mature spiritually, we will stunt our growth and stay spiritual infants forever, missing out on the privileges of adulthood. Choose today to take the steps needed to grow in your spiritual life.

Dear God, my desire is to become spiritually mature, growing more like Jesus every day. I depend upon You to lead, guide and direct my path in order to accomplish Your will in my life. Through Your Holy Spirit, please empower me to develop the areas of my life in which I need to grow closer to You and become more spiritually mature.

DAY 4: *Emotional Well-Being*

This week's memory verse states that Jesus grew in favor with God *and* with men. In order to be in good standing with our fellow humans, we need to be emotionally healthy and able to build and sustain relationships. God's influence on our hearts should be reflected in the relationships we have with others. There are many Scripture passages that relate to how God wants us to treat others.

➤ Read the following verses and in the space provided after the reference, write what each says about how we are to treat others. Then write the name of one person to whom you could apply the teaching of the verse in the blank before each reference.

- _____ Matthew 5:43-44

- _____ Matthew 5:12

- _____ Romans 12:3

- _____ Romans 12:10

- _____ Romans 12:14

- _____ Romans 12:15

- _____ Romans 12:16

- _____ Romans 12:18

The way in which we grow in favor with men is by allowing God to influence our responses to others. In doing so we reflect God's influence in our hearts. It may seem impossible to treat others in the way God has instructed us in His Word, but remember: we can do everything through Him who gives us strength (see Philippians 4:13).

Emotions often play a big part in why we overeat or make other unhealthy choices. Some people overeat (or choose unhealthy food) when they are stressed or worried, some when they are angry, hurt or sad, or even happy.

➤ What are the emotional triggers that cause you to make unhealthy choices?

➤ What can you do to choose healthy reactions to these emotional triggers?

Just as in every area of our lives, we can bring our emotions under God's control and lead well-balanced lives.

Lord God, many times I respond negatively to people without considering their feelings. I want them to see Jesus in me and to be drawn to Him by the example I set. Help me to be a good example by allowing the Holy Spirit to influence my heart in all my interactions with others.

Father, help me to deal with my emotions in healthy ways. Show me positive reactions that will keep my life in balance.

The First Place logo is a reminder to keep our lives in balance with Jesus as our focus. Let's take a closer look at it.

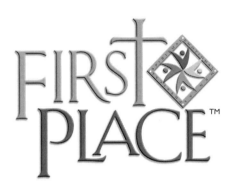
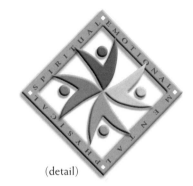

(detail)

➳ What are the four sides in the First Place logo?

➳ What does the cross at the end of "First" represent?

➳ What do you think the figure in the middle represents?

➳ In which one of the four elements do you feel the least balanced?

☐ Mentally   ☐ Spiritually

☐ Physically   ☐ Emotionally

≫ Use the following scale to mark an X on the number that best represents your overall balance right now:

1	2	3	4	5	6	7	8	9	10

Out of balance   Balanced

People tend to want instant success in a fitness program. In First Place you'll learn that just as weight gain does not happen overnight, neither will success and victory happen overnight. If you want to change your lifestyle, you must first learn to make wise choices. Allowing Jesus Christ to supply your needs and help you make the necessary changes will help you to eliminate old destructive habits and live in obedience to the life of liberty God has promised. Will you choose liberty?

Lord, I want to have total balance in my life, and I know it won't happen without You as the center of my life. I have lived in bondage for too long and I am tired of carrying old habits around. I want to be a reflection of You to others. Please help me balance my life.

DAY 6: *Reflections*

This has been a week of establishing balance in your life. Jesus maintained balance in all four areas of His life, and by keeping your focus on Him, you too can find and maintain proper balance.

Why should balance be such a big issue? In First Place you will learn that going overboard in any one area of your life can be disastrous to a healthy life. Soon, you will be pulled into the quicksand, unable to stand firmly on solid ground. "Jesus grew in wisdom and stature, and in favor with God and men" (Luke 2:52). He *grew*. Are you growing in these areas of your life?

Just as a newborn child is first nourished by milk, so a new Christian is fed milk—the foundational truth of salvation in Christ—by God until he or she is ready for solid food—a deeper, more challenging relationship with Him that changes every aspect of the believer's life (see Hebrews 5:13-14; 1 Peter 2:2-3). Perhaps you have been a Christian for a long time but have continued to subsist on spiritual milk. The foundational truths will sustain you; however, you will not experience the growth God desires for you—the growth that will change your life when you place Jesus first in every aspect of your life. Jesus taught us not to work for that which spoils but for that which endures to eternal life (see John 6:27). The four Spiritual commitments in First Place will help you to mature and balance your life in a way that is pleasing to God.

Lord Jesus, thank You for being my example of balance. Help me keep my eyes on You as I grow in maturity (see Hebrews 5:14) through a relationship with You.

Lord help me keep my eyes on You and not on the world. I want to choose that which will please You and help me grow spiritually (see 1 Corinthians 3:3).

Heavenly Father, help me desire the spiritual food that will endure throughout eternity. Create in me a hunger for that which You approve (see John 6:27).

DAY 7: *Reflections*

Being in proper balance means others can see a reflection of Jesus Christ in your life. However, old habits can creep in and thwart attempts to make good choices. Continuing destructive habits can drain your energy and create mental fatigue. Choosing to make lifestyle changes by joining First Place shows you want to drop those defeating habits and develop balance in your life, allowing God to strengthen and uplift you.

Keeping a journal during this study is one way to see God working in your life. Through writing your prayers, thoughts and insights, you will be creating a revealing account of your growth in each area of your life. Be honest and straightforward with Jesus on the pages of your journal; pour out your feelings and weaknesses, and record your victories, your learnings and your growth. If you are not the type of person who enjoys writing, consider it another opportunity to choose to do something that pleases God. He will help you come to enjoy those times of sharing on paper what is happening in your First Place journey.

Precious Savior, I want to be transformed into Your likeness—to be a reflection of You (see 2 Corinthians 3:18).

Jesus, my Lord, I know that people read me as a letter from You. As I record Your work in me on the pages of my journal, help me to be a written record of You in my daily life (see 2 Corinthians 3:3).

Lord God, help me to be strong and courageous as I learn to be obedient to You, so that in whatever I do, I will be successful (see Joshua 1:7) according to Your will.

Dear Father, help me to live a well-balanced life just as Jesus grew in wisdom and in stature and in favor with God and with men (see Luke 2:52).

Note
1. *Merriam-Webster's Collegiate Dictionary*, 10th ed., s.v. "stature."

GROUP PRAYER REQUESTS   TODAY'S DATE:_____

NAME	REQUEST	RESULTS

DOING IT ALL

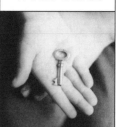

MEMORY VERSE

Be very strong and very courageous. Be careful to
obey all the law my servant Moses gave you;
do not turn from it to the right or to the left,
that you may be successful wherever you go.
Joshua 1:7

Obeying God is not multiple-choice—either we do or we don't. We cannot look at the nine First Place commitments and say, "Okay Lord, I'll attend the meetings, pray and read my Bible, but I *cannot* memorize Scripture. I'll eat according to the Live-It plan (except for French fries—You know I have to have those), but I am *not* filling out a Commitment Record (You know how busy I am). I don't mind the daily Bible study and I love calling people, but *forget* the exercise."

In this week's study, you will learn the importance of choosing to obey God in every aspect of life. Making changes in your lifestyle is not easy, but it can be done as you trust in God's abilities to help you.

DAY 1: *Horses and Chariots*

Have you ever responded to God with "But God, You know I can't do that!"? When Joshua and the Israelites were faced with a seemingly impossible situation as they faced a huge army made up of an alliance of their many enemies, "The LORD said to Joshua, 'Do not be afraid of them, because by this time tomorrow I will hand all of them over to Israel, slain. You are to hamstring their horses and burn their chariots' " (Joshua 11:6). God did as He promised when Joshua and his army defeated the enemy in spite of the odds against them.

➣ How have you seen God at work in an impossible situation?

Joshua followed God's plan even when the odds seemed against them. Choosing to obey God completely is a good choice, one that will result in victory.

➤ Which of the nine commitments are you reluctant to do as you participate in the First Place program?

➤ Why do you resist this commitment?

Many will say that it is too hard to make all of the lifestyle changes that are taught in First Place and they think they can just follow some of the commitments. This tactic might result in some positive changes, but unless you commit to following all of them, you will not see the long-lasting, life-changing results that have made First Place members victorious. It *is* difficult to change lifelong bad habits, but with God's help you *can* do it!

➤ What does Isaiah 41:10 say about how God will help you?

God is with you every step of the journey. He is there to strengthen you, help you and uphold you. Are you willing to obey His commands? Are you willing to tie up the horses that can carry you off course? Are you ready to burn the chariots of old habits? If you will trust God and do what He guides you to do, He will give you victory.

 God, help me to set aside my fears and my reluctance to follow You wholeheartedly. I ask for Your strength and help to make the right choices and follow the nine commitments for today.

DAY 2: *Nothing Spared*

One way to make choosing wisely easier in the First Place program is to inventory your kitchen, eliminating foods that may be an obstacle. This is an ongoing process, but as you replace unhealthy foods with nutritious ones, new eating habits can evolve.

➣ List some foods you need to eliminate from your kitchen.

Are there any items that you may be tempted to hang on to just in case or that you might want to hide for emergency days? Joshua 11:11 says, "They totally destroyed them, not sparing anything that breathed, and he burned up Hazor itself." If we want to be successful in making healthy lifestyle changes, we must get rid of those things that would hinder us.

➣ Are there other things in your life that take your time away from the important things? List them.

➣ What could (or should) you replace these things with?

As we become obedient, God will give us the strength, moment by moment, to do what must be done and continue on to victory.

According to John 3:16, God spared nothing in sending His one and only Son to die on the cross to pay for the sins of the world. God gave us everything He had because He loves each one of us just as we are, no matter what we do, or don't do, or how much we weigh.

Romans 12:1-2 says, "Therefore, I urge you, brothers, in view of God's mercy, to offer your bodies as living sacrifices, holy and pleasing to God—this is your spiritual act of worship. Do not conform any longer to the pattern of this world, but be transformed by the renewing of your mind. Then you will be able to test and approve what God's will is—his good, pleasing and perfect will." God spared nothing for us to live victoriously.

⟫ How can you offer your body to God as a living sacrifice?

⟫ What choices do you need to make to rid your life of all that offends God and destroys His holy temple—your body?

By *not* conforming to the world's standards, whether in entertainment, food or any other choices, you are being gradually transformed into the person God meant for you to be all along.

⟫ Can you say with assurance, "God gave His only Son to pay for my sins"? If so, how will that make a difference in the way you live today?

⟫ Write a prayer, expressing what Jesus' death on the cross means to you.

DAY 3: *Capturing the Kings*

The last part of Joshua 11:17 reads, "He captured all their kings and struck them down, putting them to death." What enemy "kings" reign in your life? It's possible for food to rule your life. When you face difficult times, do you run to the throne of chocolate, potato chips or pizza for comfort? Other kings—television, computers, shopping, worry, etc.—might be stealing precious time that could be spent in prayer, Bible study, exercise or time with family and friends.

> What kings have slipped in to ruling your life—in the place of the King of kings?

> Dethroning requires three steps as listed in Joshua 11:17.

1. He _____ all their kings

2. And _____ them down

3. Put them to _____

Capturing them can be difficult. Unhealthy foods can be disguised as the gifts or best intentions of friends or family members. Television or computer kings might be disguised as educational or necessary to keep informed. Busyness kings can wear the guise of doing good things for the Lord—when in reality it is an excuse to avoid the really important things.

Once captured, the second step is to strike them down. Knock the crown off immediately and render the king helpless. Knock those unhealthy foods off your shopping list. Turn off the television or computer and get outdoors. Let the answering machine get the mealtime and family-time calls. Drop some less-important activities to reclaim your kingdom for the Lord!

➤ List some changes you will make in order to dethrone the kings in your life.

After capturing and striking down the kings, put them to death. The Lord commanded Joshua to totally destroy the kings. Are you prepared to make lifestyle changes that will eliminate the kings in your life?

Learning to shop, cook and eat differently will put to death the old habits that helped put on the pounds. Limiting television, telephone and computer usage will provide time for physical activity or Bible study and prayer.

 O God, You are a holy and a jealous God (see Joshua 24:19) who wants to be King in my life and will not tolerate other kings. Help me be strong enough to capture, strike down and put to death any enemy king that I have allowed to replace You on the throne of my life.

DAY 4: *Complete Obedience*

According to 1 Corinthians 10:13, when we are tempted, God calls us to make wise choices and be obedient, and He will provide what we need to stand up under the temptation. We are also reminded in Scripture (see 1 Corinthians 3:16-17; 6:19-20; 2 Corinthians 6:16) that our body is His temple which was bought with a price and where the Holy Spirit resides. When we are tempted to make a bad choice, God will communicate His desire to us. Then it is up to us to choose whether or not to obey Him.

➤ What are some circumstances or situations in your life that you feel prevent you from complete obedience to the First Place program?

God knows you better than you know yourself and will not ask you to do anything beyond what you are capable of.

➭ What is something in your life that you feel is too difficult for you to give up or that you are not capable of doing?

Lay your pen down for a moment and pray, giving these situations to God. Ask Him to show you how to make changes that will enable you to keep your First Place commitments.

➭ What did He lay on your heart as you prayed and listened for His answer?

The First Place program teaches healthy options that you may choose in order to reach your weight loss and fitness goals. Whether or not you fulfill the nine commitments remains your choice. The commitments you make are between you and God.

As we learned yesterday, there are often many kings in our lives, including schedules and circumstances. We get so busy doing good things or becoming workaholics, never realizing these things have become kings. Complete obedience to God, *the* King, is the only sure way to destroy the enemy kings. A schedule that does not allow time for self-care priorities is an enemy king. Self-care includes eating healthy meals, exercising, praying, resting and spending time with family and friends.

In your journal, keep a log of how you spend your time for several days—then present it to God. Ask Him to show you how to be obedient to the commitments you made as you began your journey in First Place.

 Father, help me to recognize the counterfeit kings that usurp my time with You. Guide me to make wise choices in how I spend my time. May what I do today be honoring to You and healthy for me.

DAY 5: *Rest from the War*

Moving into the Promised Land and gaining victory in battle were not easy tasks for the Israelites. As recorded in the book of Joshua, it was only through God's power that Israel was able to conquer its many enemies. Joshua 11:16-23 records that after many battles the land was finally conquered, including the feared giants, the Anakites (see Numbers 13). Just as He did for the Israelites, God can turn your fears into victory and give you rest from war.

You may have tried many ways to lose weight. There are thousands of diets and programs that promise success. Most of us are weary from wandering in and out of this program and that diet, one after another. We become exhausted from the rules and dos and don'ts of each new method. We feel defeated and eventually give up. It's at this point where we need to hear the heart of Jesus as He says: "Come to me, all you who are weary and burdened, and I will give you rest" (Matthew 11:28).

Do you want to experience God's rest? When we do as God directs— all of it, in total obedience, sparing nothing—He will give us complete rest.

➤ Read the following Scriptures and write the key thoughts you find in each one:

- Exodus 20:8-11

- Joshua 1:13

- 1 Kings 5:3-4

- Matthew 11:28-30

Thank You, Lord, for loving me enough to care what happens in my life.

Thank You for the promise that You will give me rest for my soul. Help me to obediently take Your easy yoke and to allow You to help me carry my burdens.

DAY 6: *Reflections*

In this week's study we have learned that selective obedience is not truly obedience. Have you ever thought, *How can God expect me to do everything He says to do? He knows I'm not perfect.* Maybe you have told God, "But I did everything *except* . . . " God knows all of our imperfections, and He wants to teach us how the things left undone can prevent us from reaching our goals.

God sent His only Son, Jesus Christ, to die on the cross at Calvary, to pay for your sins and mine. He spared nothing, left nothing undone. Jesus paid for it all. What if God had said, "I will only allow My Son to pay for your past sins. You will have to work out the future ones on your own"? But He didn't do that. Jesus died to pay for *all* your sins—past, present and future. He did everything His Father told Him to do. Because of His total obedience, you can have eternal life in heaven with Him.

There are many Scriptures that emphasize how important total obedience is to God. Finding and memorizing them is the best way to reinforce what you have learned this week. Several are listed here, but using a concordance, you can find even more. Write a prayer using each of the following verses:

>> "Through your offspring all nations on earth will be blessed, because you have obeyed me" (Genesis 22:18).

>> "If you love me, you will obey what I command. Whoever has my commands and obeys them, he is the one who loves me. . . . If anyone loves me, he will obey my teaching" (John 14:15,21,23).

>> "Although he was a son, he learned obedience from what he suffered and, once made perfect, he became the source of eternal salvation for all who obey him" (Hebrews 5:8-9).

DAY 7: *Reflections*

Are you aware that God is a jealous God? Not jealous of you, but *for* you. He wants to be the reigning King in your life. God loves you so much and longs to spend time with you. Why? To teach you great and unsearchable things unknown to you (see Jeremiah 33:3). God won't break down your door and demand your attention. Instead, He waits for you to invite Him in (see Revelation 3:20). God doesn't want to be King on just some days in your life; He wants to be the King of your life *every day*.

Getting rid of the kings that consume time you could be spending with God involves making wise choices. Becoming aware of these other kings is the important first step in striking them down and eliminating them from your life. Knowing how much God loves you, wouldn't you want to do whatever it takes to have more time with Him? When you choose to follow God in complete obedience, you will experience His rest and peace.

What stands between you and complete obedience? Fear can prevent people from trusting. God tells us we need not fear, because He is with us (see Isaiah 41:10; Matthew 28:20; Romans 8:35-39). We need not fear our enemies because He protects us (see Psalm 27).

Rebelliousness can keep us from doing what God commands us to do. It causes defeat in our lives and is displeasing to God. When rebellion is the root of partial obedience, Satan applauds and encourages you to continue in your journey toward failure. God will defeat your enemies if you will ask Him.

My holy and righteous God, I am thankful that You are a jealous God, wanting me to love You above all things (see Exodus 20:5). Help me to eliminate anything that prevents me from loving You wholeheartedly.

Heavenly Father, I call upon You to help me with my rebellious spirit. Forgive me for not following Your commands, and create in me a desire and the power through the Holy Spirit to follow after You. Thank You for Your promise that You will not forsake me, Lord (see Deuteronomy 31:6).

O God, help me to remember that I express my love for You by obeying Your commands and that Your commands are not burdensome because everyone who is born of You overcomes the world (see 1 John 5:3-4).

Lord, help me to be strong and very courageous and to obey Your commands. Thank You for Your promise of success when I obey Your will for my life (see Joshua 1:7).

GROUP PRAYER REQUESTS TODAY'S DATE:_____

NAME	REQUEST	RESULTS

ACTION BRINGS HOPE

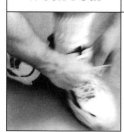

MEMORY VERSE

Therefore, prepare your minds for action;
be self-controlled; set your hope fully on
the grace to be given you when
Jesus Christ is revealed.

1 Peter 1:13

Have you ever gone through a crisis where it seems no one is doing anything to bring about resolution? Cheryl was involved in a car accident and dealt with insurance companies, agents and auto repair people. Still, her car was not being repaired as she continued to pay for a rental. Each time Cheryl called her agent she ended up in voice mail. The insurance company shuffled her from person to person. She felt powerless to do anything. She lost hope of ever getting her car fixed until she hired an attorney to write a letter to the insurance company and the agent. Her car was repaired in less than a week.

When we make contact with someone in authority, we have taken action which brings hope for a solution. In this week's study, we will learn ways to prepare for action. Preparing mentally, physically, spiritually and emotionally for action will bring hope.

DAY 1: *Prepare Your Mind*

In 1 Corinthians 9:24-27, Paul compared spiritual training with physical training for a competition. If you have ever participated in a race or competitive sporting event, you know it requires preparation of the mind as well as physical discipline. Athletes choose the grueling work of self-denial and daily disciplines of training. They also understand the necessity for mental preparation before entering the race. As you prepare yourself for action, allow God to fill your mind, replacing your thoughts with His.

➢ Describe your purpose in joining First Place.

Athletes need to understand their purpose before they can set goals for their training. It is important to clarify your purpose for joining First Place so that you know what you need to do or change.

Besides needing clearly stated goals to prepare for competitions, athletes must also get rid of self-defeating attitudes. Preparation for competition requires adapting to a new mind-set (see Romans 12:2). The old mind-set of defeat must be replaced with the knowledge that God wants you to succeed and will provide what you need to do so.

➢ What does each of the following Scriptures say about the importance of our mind-set?

- Isaiah 26:3

- Romans 8:5-6

- Romans 12:2

- Colossians 3:2

- 1 Peter 1:13

➢ What are some negative attitudes that you need to get rid of before you can move ahead toward meeting your First Place goals?

Some of us are content to be spectators, but God wants us to participate fully in this race called life. Are you still sitting up in the grandstand, watching others compete, or have you prepared yourself to enter the race and "run in such as way as to get the prize" (1 Corinthians 9:24)?

Today, choose to make it your purpose to run to win, and develop a plan of discipline so that you may obtain the prize. If we want to have victory, we must choose God's way. Pray, asking Him to help you make the right choice.

Father, replace any self-defeating attitudes that I might be holding on to with Your thoughts and desires for my life. I want to run to win and for godly disciplines to be my plan of action. Help me, now, to leave the grandstand, prepared to run and receive the heavenly prize that will last forever.

DAY 2: *Prepare Your Body*

Preparing your body for action begins with getting enough rest. Do you know how much sleep your body requires to function at its best? By allowing enough hours of sleep each night, you prepare yourself for peak performance.

➤ How does Matthew 11:28 show that God intends for us to rest?

➤ How much sleep do you get each night?

☐ Nine or more hours
☐ Seven to eight hours
☐ Five hours
☐ Less than five hours

A good night's sleep is essential for your body to heal, relax and be restored from the pressures and stress you encounter throughout the day. Most people need seven to eight hours of sleep in order to be fully rested, but if you spend eight hours tossing and turning, fretting and worrying, you will not be rested. The pressures and stresses of life can trigger worry, doubt and fear that can keep you awake. Not getting enough physical activity during the day, focusing on problems, drinking too much caffeine, depression or other factors can contribute to not sleeping well.

⋙ What are some things you can do to eliminate the stress triggers in your life that interrupt a good night's sleep?

Taking care of your physical well-being—eating balanced meals and getting enough exercise—during the day will help you to sleep better at night. Spending some time each evening in a relaxing activity will help too. Ending each day with the Lord in Bible reading and prayer is a good way to prepare for a good night's sleep. Limiting caffeine or other trigger foods or beverages in the evenings might also be helpful. If you consistently have difficulty sleeping, there may be physical causes (such as hormonal changes or chemical depression) that need to be investigated and treated by a physician.

Exercise is another way to prepare for action. The body that is not exercised deteriorates. Muscles can become atrophied, bones deteriorate and sluggishness, even depression, sets in. Regular exercise will help your body and your mind function better. It also aids your fight against heart disease, high blood pressure and high cholesterol.

First Place encourages three different kinds of physical activity: aerobic, strength and flexibility. These do not need to be done every single day, but they should be done three to five days a week.

⋙ Which of the three types of exercise do you enjoy doing now?

⋙ Which do you find difficult to do?

⇒ What can you do to include more exercise in your daily routine?

The body also requires a balanced diet to function properly. The First Place Live-It plan is ideal for preparing your body for action.

⇒ What are the three keys to preparing your body for action?

If you have not been diligent in getting enough rest, exercising regularly and maintaining a proper diet, ask God to help you make the necessary lifestyle changes.

Heavenly Father, help me to make taking care of my body a priority in my busy day. Lord, I need Your guidance in balancing my life, making time to spend with You, taking care of my physical needs and handling all my other duties. Teach me the wise use of my time and energy.

DAY 3: *Prepare Your Spirit*

Read Exodus 34:2. Developing a quiet time with God each day is perhaps the single most life-changing thing you can do to prepare yourself for action. Whether you have 5 minutes or 55 minutes, begin with the time you have available, asking God to increase it as you make time with Him the first priority.

⇒ What is your best time to spend with God?

For some, the best time to spend with God may be morning or midday. Others might find that evening or late at night is the best time. Some might even keep several appointments with the Lord throughout the day.

Some may be unable to have a morning quiet time due to early morning responsibilities, including small children who awaken early and require immediate attention. A job (or a spouse's job) may even interfere. Those who work all night may need to sleep through the majority of the morning. Some people are night owls and are more alert in the evening hours when the house is quiet. Whatever your best time of day to spend with God is, are you consistent in using that time to spend it with your heavenly Father?

➤ How do you spend your time with the Lord?

Your quiet time with God is to be special and personal. Consider it an appointment; write it on your calendar if that helps you to be consistent. Prepare for it by gathering your pen, highlighter, notebook (or your First Place journal) and Bible and keeping them all in one place. Having everything in one place, waiting for you, will simplify your daily meeting with God. Depending on the amount of time you have available, you may want to include some of the following in your meeting with God:

- Praise and worship God for who He is
- Confess sin, get right with God
- Read Scripture, letting God teach you
- Journal, recording your response to what you have read
- Talk to God about how to put into action what you have discovered
- Listen to God, meditate and wait for Him to speak
- Pray, make requests for others and for yourself and ask for guidance for your life needs

➤ What are some obstacles that keep you from having consistent and effective quiet times?

➤ List some of your goals for maintaining a daily quiet time.

Ask God to show you what is right for you. Don't get caught up in legalistic expectations. If you miss a day or only have time for a quick prayer after reading a verse or two, don't despair—do what you can, when you can. He knows your heart and what is going on in your life.

Take time right now to praise God for who He is. Then ask Him to help you prepare your spirit by having a daily quiet time.

Father, creator of heaven and Earth, I praise You and worship You. Increase my desire to meet with You daily and to learn more about You and what You desire for my life.

DAY 4: *Prepare Your Emotions*

Preparing yourself daily, through prayer and Scripture, to interact with others, will provide an open door for God to speak through you.

Do you have people in your life who rub you the wrong way? You might call them "heavenly sandpaper." How do you react to them? In Matthew 5:44, we are told to love our enemies and pray for them. One way to prepare your emotions for an encounter with people you react adversely to is by adding them to your prayer list, loving them with God's love.

➤ List three people with whom your interaction causes you to react in a negative way.

1. _____

2. _____

3. _____

How do you react to these people when they confront or irritate you? (Check all that apply.)

- ☐ Anger
- ☐ Retreating
- ☐ Depression
- ☐ Eating
- ☐ Spending
- ☐ Other _____

The Holy Spirit wants to soothe our soul when we are subjected to the arrows of others. He wants to comfort and console us by filling us with God's love. We can learn to love people God's way by looking at their hearts and seeing beyond the sandpaper surface to the real need in their lives.

➤ Read the following Scriptures and describe how Jesus reacted in each instance:

- Matthew 14:15-16

- Matthew 14:27

- Matthew 21:12-13

- Matthew 21:14-16

- Luke 13:11-12

- Luke 13:14-15

- Luke 18:35-42

- John 20:24-28

As we discover how Jesus saw people's real needs and responded, it becomes clear that we all have unmet needs that only God's love can meet. When we allow Him to love others through us, we are preparing our emotions for a new way of responding.

➤ In your journal, list several people you find difficult to love. Pray for them daily, asking God to love them through you.

 Lord Jesus, You know the people whose names I have listed and You know the things going on in their lives, as well as mine. I want to love these people unconditionally, Lord, and the only way I can do that is with Your help. Please help me see others as You see them.

DAY 5: *Grace, Faith and Hope*

Living a balanced life is not easy, especially in this hurried stressful world. It is only through God's grace that we have faith and hope.

➤ What is the source of our faith and hope, according to 1 Peter 1:18-21?

➤ How have you experienced God's grace, and how has that built up your faith and hope?

It is because of the loving grace of God and through the redemptive blood of His Son, Jesus Christ, that we can have the faith and hope needed to leave our empty way of life.

➤ Have you ever wondered if God would ever answer a certain prayer?

You must wait for God's timing and never give up hope or stop trusting Him. He has your best interests at heart and will respond according to His timing, not yours.

➺ Write 1 Peter 1:13 from memory.

This verse instructs us to prepare our minds and be self-controlled, setting our hope fully on the grace to be given when Jesus Christ is revealed. By preparing your mind for action and being self-controlled through the power of the Holy Spirit, living a holy life will become a natural part of you.

➺ Read Galatians 4:4-5. God chose you to be His child! What does that mean to you?

➺ Jesus suffered and died for you. How should that change your life?

➺ In your journal, record your thoughts regarding the title of this week's lesson, "Action Brings Hope." Review the daily lessons and jot down the things that are most helpful and meaningful to you. Share them in your small group at your next meeting.

 Lord, thank You for Your unfathomable grace, which gives me faith and hope. Help me to understand what my sin cost You and allow that knowledge to guide me to live a Christ-centered life.

DAY 6: *Reflections*

In this week's study, you have learned how to take action that brings hope. Whether it involves mental, physical, spiritual or emotional preparation, the key is to prepare for action in God's way.

God is the source of our hope. He *is* our hope! "Christ in you" is our "hope of glory" (Colossians 1:27). The Holy Spirit has been given to supply us with the power, strength and wisdom we need to choose and then follow His way. Are you accessing God's power to live your life, to make the changes you need to make? First you must ask for His power, and then you must use it!

Preparing for action begins with prayer. Reach out and up to our ultimate authority, our creator, God. Then spend time sitting at His feet so that you will learn how to live. Your daily quiet time with God will produce right results. Take time to reflect on God's Word and rest in the knowledge that He wants to help and guide you.

Most high God, help me to dwell in Your shelter and to rest in Your almighty shadow (see Psalm 91:1).

Father, help me to be prepared to preach the Word, in season and out of season, and help me to rebuke and encourage others with great patience and careful instructions (see 2 Timothy 4:2).

Lord, You have instructed me to love my enemies and pray for those who persecute me. That is hard to do, but I know I can trust You to provide the strength and power to do what You ask me to do (see Matthew 5:44).

DAY 7: *Reflections*

Have you ever observed a beautiful mountain with a glint of light reflecting from its peak? Perhaps there is a path leading to the base of the majestic mountain. Picture yourself walking briskly up that path, excitedly anticipating a meeting with God.

It is early in the morning, the air is cool and quiet with only the sound of the distant rustling of the trees. You begin to sing, "I lift up my eyes to you, to you whose throne is in heaven" (Psalm 123:1). You know that God has something important to share with you today. Getting up was a joyful act of obedience. Now, as you walk the path singing praises, you begin to understand God's love for you and His desire to spend time alone with you.

You stop on the path and lift your arms to heaven. You ask God to create in you a desire to meet with Him like this every day. He hears your prayer, and immediately you sense the excitement of the exchange of communication between you and God. You pray; He hears. He answers; you obey.

Suddenly, you recall other songs from God's Word and you continue on your path toward the mountain, singing praises as you walk.

> I will praise you, O LORD, with all my heart;
> I will tell of all your wonders.
> I will be glad and rejoice in you;
> I will sing praise to your name, O Most High (Psalm 9:1-2).

> It is good to praise the LORD and make music to your name,
>   O Most High
> to proclaim your love in the morning
> and your faithfulness at night (Psalm 92:1-2).

> Give thanks to the LORD, for he is good;
> his love endures forever (Psalm 118:1).

GROUP PRAYER REQUESTS   TODAY'S DATE:_____

NAME	REQUEST	RESULTS

A DISCERNING HEART

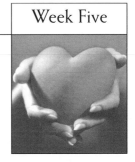

MEMORY VERSE

*So give your servant a discerning heart
to govern your people and to distinguish
between right and wrong.*

1 Kings 3:9

King Solomon, who was probably in his 20s, recognized his inability to lead the nation of Israel without God's assistance. When God came to Solomon in a dream and told him that He would give him anything he wanted, Solomon earnestly asked for a discerning heart so that he could govern God's people and distinguish between right and wrong (see 1 Kings 3:4-9).

In this week's study, we will explore how we can have a more discerning heart.

DAY 1: *Pleasing God*

When Solomon asked for wisdom, the Lord was pleased (see 1 Kings 3:10).

➤ Have you asked God for something that you knew pleased Him? What was it?

When we ask for things for the right reasons, it pleases God.

➤ Have you ever asked God for something good but wanted it for the wrong reason? What was the result?

It takes a discerning heart to ask wisely with the right motives.

➣ What does each of the following Scripture passages say about discernment?

- Proverbs 14:6

- Proverbs 15:14

- Proverbs 17:10

- Proverbs 17:24

- Philippians 1:9-10

 Lord God, like Solomon, I need Your wisdom so that I may do what is right in Your eyes. Grant me discernment in choosing the path You want me to take. I want to please You, Father, in all I say and do.

DAY 2: *Making the Right Choice*

➣ According to 1 Kings 3:11-12, how did God honor Solomon's request?

➣ Have riches, material possessions or worldly pursuits been your goal? Have you attained your goal? What has been the result?

Many times, dissatisfaction sets in after gaining the worldly things we crave. God desires much more for you than riches and material things can provide. He will shower you with many blessings.

≫ In 1 Kings 3:5, God told Solomon, "Ask for whatever you want me to give you." What would your response be if God had said that to you?

People often spend their whole lives pursuing riches, fame or power only to be dissatisfied once they acquire them. Only God can fill the deepest need within us. If you seek after God and His kingdom, He will provide for your every need.

≫ Describe something you have pursued only to feel dissatisfied after you gained it.

≫ According Proverbs 1:1-6—authored by Solomon—what is the purpose of wisdom?

≫ According to Proverbs 1:7, who despises wisdom and discipline?

≫ How has God given you wisdom and discipline in the First Place program?

➺ How does having wisdom and discipline make your life more satisfying?

Solomon prayed for wisdom, and God gave it to him, along with riches and long life (see 1 Kings 3:13-14). We are not promised riches; He gives us what we need if we put His kingdom, interests and principles first in our lives.

➺ According to Proverbs 2:9-10, what will happen when you receive wisdom from God?

Solomon asked for wisdom to carry out his job. In the First Place program, you are learning the importance of discerning between things beneficial to you, mentally, physically, spiritually and emotionally, and things that will hinder you in these areas. God wants to express His pleasure toward you just as He did with Solomon.

➺ In your journal, write what you would like God to give you, and how it would benefit you. Pray about what you have written. Then, spend time listening for Him to speak in response to your request.

 Heavenly Father, You know my deepest desire and my reason for wanting to see it fulfilled. I pray that You will align my thoughts with Yours and I would only seek Your will for my life.

DAY 3: *Receiving Riches and Honor*

God loves His children so much, and wants to shower them with blessings. His resources are unlimited as He looks for opportunities to bless you with gifts you never dreamed of having (see 1 Kings 3:13-14). God requires only that we be obedient to Him and walk in His ways. The benefits that result from obedience will bless your life.

➤ What gifts did God give Solomon that Solomon did not ask for (v. 13)?

➤ If God values discernment more than riches and honor, why do you believe He granted Solomon things that Solomon did not ask for?

In Matthew 6:33-34, Jesus tells us not to worry about our life. If we put Him first in our life, we will be given all we need. Putting Christ first in your life does not mean simply praying first thing each day. It means seeking Him first when you need guidance, protection or comfort. It means following His will for your life.

➤ In what ways have your desires and lifestyle changed since you have been in First Place?

There is a huge difference between planning for tomorrow and worrying about it. Productive planning means setting goals, taking steps and trusting God. Planning in this way helps to alleviate worry.

➤ Describe how you have planned for the future in one area of your life.

When you worry, you are consumed with fears and doubts that God can handle the problem. Soon the worries about tomorrow affect your relationship with God today.

❧ Describe a time when you allowed worry to interfere with your relationship with God. What was the result of the situation? What lesson did you learn?

Putting Christ first in our life and trusting Him completely is our assurance that our life will be on track. We cannot even begin to know the many gifts and blessings that await us in the future. God wants to provide for us and help us enjoy a bountiful life. Worry and doubt are dead ends. Trust and obedience are the paths to enjoying God's promises for your future.

 God Almighty, I give You thanks for Your many blessings, for all the eternal riches and honor You have given to me already. I pray, Father, that You will help me to put Christ first in my life, relying on Him to take care of my every need.

DAY 4: Attaining Long Life

❧ What is the promise God gave to Solomon in 1 Kings 3:14? What is the big "if" in this promise?

❧ How does God's promise to Solomon relate to Matthew 6:33?

❧ What areas of the First Place program are you having difficulty fulfilling?

≫ Why do you think you are having difficulty in these areas?

The nine commitments of the First Place program are tools that will enable you to walk in His ways, obeying His statutes and commands.

Commitment number two is prayer. Praying daily will help you give Christ first place in your life.

≫ List several needs you have right now.

Commitment three is Scripture reading. By choosing passages from the Old and New Testaments, you will be enlightened on how God deals with His children.

≫ Write down two Scripture references that you will read and reflect on today.

1. _____

2. _____

Memorizing a verse a week is the fourth commitment. Hiding God's Word in your heart will give you the tools you need to fight temptation.

≫ Write this week's verse from memory.

The last of the spiritual commitments is Bible study. If you devote time daily to your Bible study, you will learn to follow the path God has set for you.

≫ Write down two of the truths you have learned so far this week.

1. _____

2. _____

Your First Place leader wants to help you. Share with him or her any difficulties you are experiencing. Ask your group for prayer and support as you seek God's help to overcome the obstacles to your success. One of the biggest blessings of following God and obeying His statutes and commands is a healthier, more enjoyable life. Along with your spiritual commitments to follow God, eating wisely and exercising regularly are tangible ways you can cooperate with God to improve the quality of your life.

 Heavenly Father, my commitment to You is important to me, and I need Your help to overcome the obstacles that get in my way. Help me to walk in Your ways by obeying Your statutes and commands. I want to have a healthy life, but even more, I desire to please You in everything I do.

DAY 5: *Receiving Measureless Blessings*

Not only did God give Solomon wisdom and very great insight, but also a breadth of understanding as measureless as the sand on the seashore—the wisest man of his time (see 1 Kings 4:29-34). There was no limit to the blessings God gave to Solomon.

➤ What kind of insight and understanding do you wish you possessed in dealing with your weight and/or health problems?

Solomon spoke 3,000 proverbs and composed 1,005 (see 1 Kings 4:32). Each week you are asked to memorize a Scripture verse. How are you doing with your memory verses? If you have difficulty memorizing, try writing the verse several times each day or team up with someone in your group to help each other memorize your verses. The encouragement you can give each other will go a long way in all aspects of your life.

➤ Write this week's memory verse (without looking!).

✎ Name some blessings God has provided for you since you began this session of First Place.

Dear God, I am willing to do all that You ask me to do. Help me be consistent and follow Your direction for my life. Thank You for Your measureless blessings, Lord. I praise You and worship You.

DAY 6: *Reflections*

A discerning heart is a valuable thing to have. You have learned this week that by being discerning you can please God and make right choices. God wants you to enjoy an abundant life, and the way to do that is to make wise choices.

Having a discerning heart can help you know God better and develop a closer relationship with Him. It will give you understanding of the meaning of obedience. Think about what having a discerning heart can do for you in other areas of your life, your family, church and career. We begin by wanting to please God. When we ask for the right things and for the right reasons, He blesses us abundantly and provides so much more than we asked for.

Precious Lord, I need the knowledge that comes only to the discerning heart (see Proverbs 14:6).

Father God, help me to live to please You. Give me the discernment to do so consistently (see 1 Thessalonians 4:1).

Heavenly Father, sometimes I've asked for things for the wrong reasons. Please change my heart so that my only motive is to please You (see James 4:3).

DAY 7: *Reflections*

Your life, like Solomon's, can be full of blessings. The reservoir of spiritual resource in the proverbs and songs Solomon wrote must have helped greatly in the valleys he walked (see 1 Kings 4:32). It is in the valleys that we cry out for help, direction and rescue. How many Scriptures do you know by heart that would help you through a dark valley? Remember: You cannot recall that which you do not know.

As of this session, you have learned five memory verses. The memory verses have been set to music to help you retain them more easily. If you are still having trouble memorizing Scripture, tell your First Place leader and ask for help in your group meeting. Most of all, *ask God* to help you memorize His precious Word. That will please Him, and He will bless you abundantly in response.

Father, I want to delight in the Your law and meditate on it day and night (see Psalm 1:2).

I will praise You, O Lord, with all my heart. I will sing Your praise and I will praise Your name for Your love and faithfulness (see Psalm 138:1-2).

Thank You that "what is impossible with men is possible with God" (Luke 18:27). When I am discouraged in following You wholeheartedly, help me to remember that You will help me accomplish the seemingly impossible.

Father God, give me a discerning heart to govern my affairs and to distinguish between right and wrong (see 1 Kings 3:9).

GROUP PRAYER REQUESTS   TODAY'S DATE:_____

NAME	REQUEST	RESULTS

EVERYTHING PERMISSIBLE

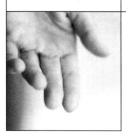

MEMORY VERSE

"Everything is permissible for me"—
but not everything is beneficial.
"Everything is permissible for me"—
but I will not be mastered by anything.
1 Corinthians 6:12

Christ has set us free. We are to live in freedom from the multitude of man-made religious rules, but we should not use our freedom as an excuse to sin. Learning to live as free people takes time and practice. As we continue on our First Place journey, we will discover that although everything is permissible, not everything is good for us.

In this week's study, we will learn how to choose the things that are most helpful to maintaining the healthy, abundant life that God wants for us.

DAY 1: *Balanced*

Jesus instructed that if we hold to His teachings, we are really His disciples. Only then will we know the truth that sets us free (see John 8:31-32). However, in our freedom we need guidance to help us stay on track.

The memory verse for this week states that everything is permissible, but not everything is helpful. Let's examine each of the four areas of our lives, keeping in mind the question: *Is this helpful?*

➤ Mentally—List one TV program you watched last week, one audio-tape/CD you listened to and one magazine you read. Next to each item, write one way the item stretched your mind and helped you grow.

- TV program

- Audiotape/CD

- Magazine

➤ Physically—Consider the following three areas. Did your recent (today or yesterday) choice in each area provide your body with the energy and nutrients necessary for good health?

- Food choice(s)

- Exercise

- Rest

➤ Spiritually—Have you read a motivational book, heard a spiritual message, discussed something with family or friends, or done something similar recently?

- How did this activity point you to Jesus?

- In what way did this activity strengthen your faith?

- How did this activity benefit God's kingdom?

- How pleasing do you think this activity was to the Lord?

➤ Emotionally—Think about a family member or friend who has irritated you recently. Write down your response to that person's action, using the following questions:

- Was your reaction helpful or harmful to the relationship? In what way?

- Did your reaction build up or injure the other person or yourself? How?

- Did your reaction honor God? Describe how it did or didn't.

 Thank You, God, for the freedom You have given me. I know I'm responsible for making wise choices, and I need Your direction and help to hold to Your teachings. When I am tempted to make an unwise decision, please allow Your Holy Spirit to intervene and show me the right way to respond.

DAY 2: *Who Controls Whom*

Having been set free by Christ, we are cautioned not to allow ourselves to be burdened again by a yoke of slavery (see Galatians 5:1).

➤ Are there certain foods, actions or habits that still call your name and pull you back into slavery? List them.

" 'Everything is permissible for me'—but I will not be mastered by anything" (1 Corinthians 6:12). Do certain foods or activities still hold you in their power? Don't fear these things; rather, deal with them and regain control.

If a candy bar, anger or shopping spree is calling your name and you know the power it used to have over you, take control immediately. Take a stand, asking yourself, *Who controls whom?* Ignoring, indulging or encouraging the temptation draws you into its power.

➣ Name some things that still have power over you. How do you deal with them presently? How should you deal with them in the future?

Name It	Dealt with in the Past	Deal with in the Future

When we allow something to control or master us, we become a slave to it (see 2 Peter 2:19). With God as our master, we will not give in to harmful temptations.

 God, help me live and walk in the freedom You have given me. Please free me from [name the things] and strengthen me to stand firm.

DAY 3: *Your Body Is His Temple*

In today's society, there are many who feel they have the right to do whatever they want with their own body. As a Christian, you have the Holy Spirit living within you; therefore, your body is no longer yours to do with as you please because it is His temple (see 1 Corinthians 6:19).

➣ What does 1 John 2:16-17 say will happen to the world and its desires?

➣ What will happen to those who do the will of God?

Claiming ownership of your body may seem like freedom, but the childish "it's-mine-to-do-with-as-I-want" attitude is truly enslavement to fleshly desires.

➣ Describe one of your own it's-mine attitudes regarding your body.

➣ Scripture states that God owns our bodies. Read 1 Corinthians 6:19 and fill in the missing words.

Do you not know that your _____ is a

_____ of the _____ , who is

in you, whom you have received from God? You are not your

_____.

Consider your body as a building dedicated to the worship of God.

➣ If you owned a beautiful mansion, what types of furnishings would you choose to put in it?

➣ Knowing your body is a beautiful temple of the Lord, what kinds of foods and activities would be appropriate for it?

➣ According to Romans 12:1, why are we to offer our bodies as a living sacrifice to God?

➤ Offering your body as a living sacrifice is a spiritual act of worship. What are some practical ways that you can offer your body as a living sacrifice.

 Precious Lord, I know my body is the temple where the Holy Spirit resides. I want Your temple to be a place of honor, worthy for You to call home. Show me what I need to do today and the rest of the week to make my body a place fit for worship.

DAY 4: *Bought and Paid For*

Many early Christians were slaves. There are some countries today that still either practice or allow the buying and selling of humans into slavery. However, all people are slaves to sin unless they have accepted Christ's gift of salvation (see John 8:34-36). The only One who has the power to conquer sin and set us free is Jesus because of His death on the cross in our place. Wherever the practice of slavery has been abolished, owners no longer have any power over their former slaves. When we become Christians, the power sin had in our lives can no longer bind us. Becoming a slave to Christ means we have been freed from our bondage to sin and given eternal life by Him (see Romans 6:22-23).

➤ According to 1 Corinthians 7:23, you were bought at a great price. What price was paid for your freedom?

➤ What does it mean to you to be free from sin?

The death of God's only Son was the price paid. Because such a high price was paid, you now belong to Christ. When you became a slave to Christ, you were set free from sins of all kinds (see Romans 6:17-18). Just as Christ values you because He paid such a high price through His death, you should place great value on your body.

➤ What is something you bought for a high price and that you treasure dearly?

➤ What kind of care do you give it?

A friend of mine once purchased an antique Wedgwood bowl and pitcher set. She paid a high price for it and it belongs to her. She has placed it on an antique washstand where she can enjoy its beauty. She would never fill it with trash, but she protects it from damage. She values it so much that she takes special care of it.

Thank You, Lord for freeing me from the bondage of sin. I know I now belong to You and that You value and take care of me. You've given me freedom of choice and will not barge into my life without permission. Today, I give You permission to help me care for my body properly.

DAY 5: *Honoring God with Your Body*

God owns your body, and you should use it to give glory to Him (see 1 Corinthians 6:20). When you talk, your speech should be wholesome, uplifting and beneficial. When you work with your hands, in whatever labor you do, your work should reflect the One you are committed to. Everything you do, whether in word or deed, should be done in the name of Jesus (see Colossians 3:17).

➣ Listed below are several ways you can honor God with your body. Check which side of your life it represents (the first is done for you). Add two activities of your own that you have done today.

How Honored	Mental	Physical	Spiritual	Emotional
Interact well				X
Exercise regularly				
Read worthwhile books				
Memorize Scripture				
Lead a Bible study				
Learn a new skill				

Honoring God with your body shows the world that you have put Christ first place in your whole life. How you dress, talk, do business, socialize and maintain your health speaks clearly of the quality of your relationship with Christ. Actions and attitudes speak more loudly than your words.

Some people think they are honoring God by attending church, tithing and serving on countless committees, yet at work (or even home), they treat others unfairly, repeatedly display impatience or anger, or they're destroying their own health by drinking, smoking, overeating or using drugs. These actions dishonor God's temple and His name.

➣ In what area of your life might you be dishonoring God?

➣ According to Titus 2:11-13, what are we to say no to?

➣ How are we to live?

Christ gave Himself for us. It is our responsibility to do what is right and to honor Him.

Lord Jesus, I want to honor You in every way and every day, in all four areas of my life. Show me today how I can begin to honor You with my body.

DAY 6: *Reflections*

We experience a real sense of power when we say no to something that is permissible but not beneficial. *Who controls whom?* is a question we must ponder when facing difficult choices or temptations. Are you mastered by a bad habit? Is there a particular food that always seems to call your name? Perhaps there is a person in your life who seems to control your emotions. Think about how it would feel to remove that habit from your life and replace it with something that would reflect Christ in you. How would it make you feel to look at that emotion/food/action that haunts and taunts you and say, "Out you go—out of my sight and mind"? Would you feel free if you were able to unshackle yourself from people who try to control your life? You *can* do it, for you can do everything through Him who gives you strength (see Philippians 4:13).

You can choose to use God's power to regain control and free yourself from those things or habits that have enslaved you. It is all about choosing who your master will be: sin or God. With God as the master of your life, you are free from slavery to sin. In First Place, you are not told "You cannot have this or that." Instead, you learn to make wise choices.

Dear Lord, I want *You* as the master of my life, guiding me as I stand strong in the face of temptation (see Romans 14:4).

Thank You Lord, that I have been set free from sin. I am thankful that because You gave your life for me, I can have eternal life (see Romans 6:22).

Lord Jesus, help me to stand firm in times of temptation and say no to things that would gain power over me (see Ephesians 6:14).

DAY 7: *Reflections*

Thinking of your body as a temple of the Lord may be scary or humbling. How pleased God is when His temple is being well cared for and maintained as a valuable vessel available for His use! When you choose to be properly rested, you will be restored physically, mentally, emotionally and spiritually. Yes, you can stay up late, crowd your mind with television, ignore Bible study and fill your body with junk, but why would you want to destroy God's temple? The benefits of choosing wisely are so great.

God desires the best for you, and throughout His Word He encourages you to make wise choices. He is pleased to reside in a temple fit for a king—*the* King. Is your temple fit for the King of kings? If not, God is waiting to help you get it under control. It is not just the outside that should look suitable for His holy temple, but the inside where the Holy Spirit dwells must be suitable too.

Some things that fill our minds can be ugly and displeasing to God. When we allow unfit reading material or TV programs to filter in, they leave a bad residue and can cloud our ability to make wise choices. Junk food is aptly named. Junk doesn't belong in the holy temple of the Lord. Allowing emotions to rule our lives will cause no end of sorrow and trouble, damaging our relationships and causing physical problems as well.

Physical inactivity will destroy our bodies from the inside out, causing loss of muscle, reducing heart and lung capacity, and rendering us unable to be on the move for God. Spiritual idleness—absence of time spent with the Lord in worship and prayer, Bible study and memorizing Scripture—can cause a Christian's heart to grow cold.

Take inventory of how you are treating your temple. Do some temple cleaning and make it a place—both inside and out—in which God will be pleased to dwell.

Father God, I am so thankful that Your Holy Spirit lives in me. I want my temple to be truly fit for the master of my life (see 1 Corinthians 3:16).

God of heaven, You live and work in and through me. You are my God and my body is Your temple. Help me keep it pure (see 2 Corinthians 6:16).

Lord Jesus, I know You paid a great price for me and I am not my own, but Yours. I want to honor You with my body (see 1 Corinthians 6:20).

Dear Lord, help me to remember that " 'everything is permissible for me'—but not everything is beneficial. 'Everything is permissible for me'—but I will not be mastered by anything" (1 Corinthians 6:12). Thank You for the freedom I have in You, and give me the wisdom to make right choices.

GROUP PRAYER REQUESTS   TODAY'S DATE:_____

NAME	REQUEST	RESULTS

REBUILDING YOUR LIFE

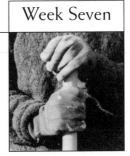

MEMORY VERSE

Unless the LORD *builds the house,*
its builders labor in vain.

Psalm 127:1

First Place is not an overnight fad for quick weight loss; it is a lifestyle change. God expects us to cooperate with Him as He works at rebuilding our lives. He empowers, enables and encourages, but we must put forth effort to accomplish goals so that He may take pleasure in our success and be honored by it. What better pleasure and honor to God than to have a person be transformed mentally, physically, spiritually and emotionally?

You are now over halfway through this First Place study. If you feel that you are not achieving all the goals you have set, let this be an evaluation and rebuilding time. If you feel you are on track with your goals, let this be a time for you to reaffirm and refine your commitment to make wise choices. In this week's study, we will learn from the prophet Haggai the steps we can take to rebuild our life just as he led the people of Jerusalem in rebuilding the ruined Temple.

- 🍎 Give careful thought to your ways.
- 🍎 Get up.
- 🍎 Gather the tools.
- 🍎 Build the temple.

DAY 1: *Careful Thought*

If you were planning to build a home, one of the first steps to take would be to meet with an architect to discuss your ideas and draw up plans. The entire process would be carefully thought through before any materials were ordered. When building a healthier lifestyle, it is equally important to give careful thought to the life you are trying to build.

In Haggai 1:7, the Lord says, "Give careful thought to your ways." It is interesting to note that the phrase "give careful thought" is repeated four times in this short two-chapter book! The Jews were about to embark on an overwhelming task of rebuilding the Temple out of the ruins of the original. Think back over the previous weeks, evaluating your previous Commitment Records, to answer the following questions:

➣ List those things that you have been doing right.

➣ List the things you should have been doing but chose not to do.

In rebuilding your life, you must meet with God, the great architect, and go over His plans for you. God knows the things you need to be doing but are choosing not to do. If you will ask Him to show you what those things are and ask for His help in doing them, He is ready and willing to help you. After all, you are His temple, whether you need some refurbishing or rebuilding!

➣ List some things that you knew would not be beneficial to your body, but chose to do anyway.

Everything you do has a consequence. The wise decisions you make will bless you; the unwise decisions will not. Numbers 32:23 says, "You may be sure that your sin will find you out." When we are disobedient to what God has shown us to do, or not to do, we are sinning—and our sins will find us out.

✏ Consider how you answered the previous questions. Describe the effects these unwise choices have had on your progress up to now.

 Lord God, I have sinned by my disobedience and need Your forgiveness. I know You have advised me when I faced temptation and times of confusion, but often I didn't heed Your advice. I have felt the consequences and I humble myself before You. I am committing myself to following Your direction. Thank You for Your love. I receive the forgiveness You so graciously give.

DAY 2: *Get Going*

Haggai was a prophet who, along with Zechariah, encouraged the returning Jewish exiles to rebuild the Temple which had laid in ruins for many years. The exiles were overwhelmed at the enormity of the task and were using any excuse they could find not to begin the rebuild. Haggai admonished them in Haggai 1:2-11.

Overwhelming projects can cause a person to become immobile, unwilling to try to tackle the mountain of work that needs to be done. The temptation is to shrug it off as impossible and give up before you have begun. Instead of giving up, take your projects to God. When tackling large jobs, you must first make sure your relationship with God is the cornerstone of the project. Once you have done that, get up and begin! God will supply the strength and power necessary to get the work done.

✏ Describe a situation in which you felt unable to reach your goal and so just stopped trying. (For instance, paying off debts, cleaning up a disorganized house or losing weight.)

❧ Haggai told the people in the beginning of verse 8 to "go up into the mountains." How does this relate to your seemingly impossible task?

Often we look at the big job and feel overwhelmed. Overwhelming jobs can be called "goal stoppers" because they are obstacles in your attempt to rebuild your life. When we look only at the big picture, we can begin to feel that our goal is unreachable.

After giving careful thought to what you have or have not done up to this point, the second step in the rebuilding process is to get going. Just getting up breaks the inertia and prepares our body, mind, spirit and emotions for action.

If credit cards or other extensive debt has overwhelmed you, perhaps the first step may be to cut up the cards to avoid adding to what you already owe. After doing that, you can contact the creditors or a credit-counseling agency to work out a payment plan to pay off the existing debt.

Perhaps you have neglected to keep your home organized, allowing junk mail to pile up, important papers to become lost and clutter to take over. Your first step might be to clean off one countertop or organize one drawer or closet. Begin small, and once you achieve success with that area, move to the next. Focus your attention on only one area at a time and avoid looking at the bigger picture of what needs to be done.

If being overweight has shackled you, you've already taken the first step in becoming a member of the First Place program. Each week's lesson will yield new truths to help you move toward your goal. Consider what your next step must be. Perhaps you need to stop bringing junk food into your home. Maybe you can start walking a mile, increasing your distance or pace a little each week.

❧ What is the first step you will choose to take on your way to over-coming your goal stopper?

Don't try to change everything at once. Pick one thing that you will commit to doing this week. Pray right now asking God to show you how to begin. Listen as He speaks to you and be encouraged as you begin the rebuilding process in whatever area God is showing you.

≫ In your prayer journal, write down an insight you gained from your prayer time.

 Dear Lord, I don't know where to begin. I have hit a goal stopper head-on and can't seem to get past it. You know the overwhelming weight of what I am facing. I know You possess the power and strength to lift this heavy burden from me. I am willing to get up and do whatever You tell me to do. Let me know where You want me to begin.

DAY 3: *Gather Tools*

Haggai 1:8 says, "Bring down timber." The people were instructed to gather the materials necessary to build the Temple. They had been so busy thinking about themselves—having enough to eat, clothes to wear and money—that they forgot about building God's temple (see Haggai 1:5-6). Now the time had come for the Temple to be built, and the people were told to go into the mountains and gather the materials.

The First Place program teaches us to put Christ first in our lives. Building a relationship with Him must take priority over everything else. Once your relationship with Jesus is built, you can use the First Place materials and tools to rebuild God's temple: you!

≫ Have you established a personal relationship with Jesus?

☐ Yes   ☐ No

If you haven't established a personal relationship with Jesus, there is no better time than right now! If you do not know how, turn to page 29 in your *First Place Member's Guide* and read "Steps to Becoming a Christian." Or call your First Place leader or another member and ask him or her to help you become a member of God's family. Once you have taken this step, share your decision with a Christian friend or group member so that you will receive the encouragement you deserve for making the most important choice of your life!

If you have already accepted Christ as your Savior, it is time to begin (or continue) rebuilding. The Live-It plan along with the other eight commitments are tools to help you rebuild your life—inside and out.

➤ When you think about rebuilding your life, which area of rebuilding do you find most overwhelming?

➤ What tools, material or resources do you *already have* to begin the rebuilding of that area?

➤ What tools, material or resources do you *lack* to begin the rebuilding of that area?

➤ Where will you get the necessary tools, materials or resources? Who can help you in gathering them?

Procrastination was the enemy of God's temple builders. Waiting for the right time or until you have everything lined up, just so, will hamper your chances of experiencing victory. God will meet you right where you are to help you get started, and He will be with you throughout the process. He will not desert you, but will see you through to victory (see Haggai 1:13; 2:4).

This week we have learned to plan, get going and gather our tools. Are you ready? Have you taken these first three steps? If not, take time now to go back, review and apply them. Don't put it off another day.

➺ In your prayer journal, list each step you need to take and how you have prepared for it. Be specific and detailed. Submit these to God and ask Him to help you follow through.

 Father, I lay out my plans before You and ask for Your help in taking the first step. I have established my relationship with You and want to work with You in rebuilding my life. Thank You, Lord, for being there for me.

DAY 4: *Build the Temple*

It is easy to become discouraged when you feel you are the only one working on a large project. Left to yourself, doubt, discouragement and fear may set in. The work seems more difficult; progress slows and may stop altogether. That's why First Place is especially successful in a small-group setting. The support of the group is a source of encouragement as you share your struggles with others.

➺ According to Ephesians 2:19-22, who is involved in building God's temple?

The whole building is joined together and rises to become a holy temple in the Lord; and in Him you, too, are being built together to become a dwelling where God lives by his Spirit.

➺ How does it feel, knowing you are not alone in the rebuilding of your body, the temple of the Lord?

We are joined with God's people in the First Place program world-wide. We support one another in prayer. We also provide encouragement, give help and share information when needed.

➤ How does being a part of First Place encourage you to rebuild your temple?

Now is the time to build. Do not wait for Monday or the first of the month. Jesus Christ is the cornerstone that has already been laid. You can begin rebuilding now! Remember there are many people available to help you when you are discouraged or you need strengthening.

 Heavenly Father, I am ready to build. I'm thankful that I'm not alone in the building process. I am thankful for Your strength and guidance. I'm excited that we are being built together and that Your Holy Spirit lives in me. Help me to do my part Lord, and do the work You ask me to do.

Remind me, Lord, to be an encourager to others in my First Place group.

DAY 5: *Greater Glory and Peace*

After months of remodeling their home, our neighbors could not believe how bright and beautiful it looked compared to the "before" pictures. They had given a lot of careful thought and planning to the project. They got busy, gathered workers and materials, and rebuilt their old house into the beautiful home they had dreamed of for years. They had saved their resources in preparation for the task, and once the rebuilding was done, they felt peace within the walls of their newly rebuilt home.

God will provide all the resources we need to rebuild our lives.

➤ What does the end of Haggai 1:8 say about God's purpose in wanting the Temple rebuilt?

➤ How does (or should) giving pleasure and honor to God by building a healthy temple affect your goals in First Place?

➤ What does Haggai 2:9 mean to you concerning meeting your First Place goals?

We are working with God, under His direction, to rebuild our body— His temple. By using God's tools and resources, we are guaranteed He will complete the work and it will be top notch (see Philippians 1:6). When you live in obedience to God, you develop a standard of living that will last a lifetime. The principles that you learn from God's Word will help you change unhealthy habits into the right way of living. Lifestyle changes will occur as you memorize Scripture to call upon in hard times.

➤ What are some ways you can help make your new body better than the former?

When our bodies are out of control, our lives are chaotic. Out-of-control eating can spill into other areas of our lives, causing frustration, upheaval and confusion.

➤ Read Haggai 2:9 and fill in the missing word.

"And in this place I will grant _____," declares the LORD Almighty.

➤ God wants to give you peace in your rebuilt temple. The following verses provide insight into the peace God wants you to have. After reading each one, write down the insight that God gives you.

- John 14:27

- 1 Corinthians 14:33a

- Ephesians 2:13-15

- Philippians 4:6-7

- 2 Thessalonians 3:16

By making peace with us through His blood, shed on the cross, Jesus reconciled all things to Himself (see Colossians 1:19-20). When we turn our lives over to Him, we are reconciled to Him and His Holy Spirit dwells in us—His temple.

 God Almighty, creator of all things, thank You for Your provision for my peace. Thank You for my new self, free from the burden of sin and free to choose to love You. I will honor You with my body and give You the praise and glory for all You have done for me.

DAY 6: *Reflections*

Many couples plan their dream house for years, giving careful thought to all the features and the look they desire. They plan mentally for how they will approach the project, who will be hired, what materials they will use and which furnishings they will select. They budget carefully and detail their plans. Often the blueprints will have to be revised several times, and new ideas will replace those that were not suitable to the finished project.

As you seek to rebuild your house—God's temple—giving careful thought is even more important than building an earthly dwelling place. God cautions you to plan carefully. Rebuilding is necessary because of bad choices made in the past. God wants to help you—He will meet you where you are right now. It doesn't matter what bad habits rule your life or how much you weigh; He will begin right where you are and help you rebuild from the inside out. He will help you change your poor habits and teach you to make wise choices in order to transform your body into a beautiful temple. God will be your architect, material supplier and coworker as He will accomplish His purpose in you—with your cooperation.

Father God, I want to work with You to rebuild Your temple—my body. Help me to be the fellow worker I need to be (see 1 Corinthians 3:9).

Thank You, God, that we are joined together, and we are raising a holy temple in You (see Ephesians 2:21).

DAY 7: *Reflections*

Procrastination is an enemy of the Lord. It stops Christians from moving forward to accomplish God's purpose in their lives. Sometimes a project seems overwhelming when you look at all that needs to be done. Instead of beginning, you put off doing the things that will carry you to victory. The words, "someday," "later" and "after a while" creep into your vocabulary. Soon the project is abandoned and you feel like a failure.

We've learned this week that God says, "Get up!" Today, take the first step toward your goal. Do one thing—the first thing that God tells you to do. As long as you remain immobile, God's temple cannot be rebuilt. You will not wake up tomorrow morning and suddenly find that you are thin, out of debt or organized. Every goal you set takes planning, preparation and hard work. But God is here to help you every step of the way: " 'Be strong, . . . and work. For I am with you,' declares the LORD Almighty" (Haggai 2:4).

God may direct you to begin a walking program or take swimming lessons. He may lead you to set up a budget and start tithing. If you follow Him in obedience and don't put off the first day toward victory, you will experience blessings beyond your imagination. Remember: Procrastination is an obstacle to reaching your destination.

 Lord, just as the children of Israel responded to Moses when he gave them Your words, so I do too: "Everything the LORD has said we will do" (Exodus 24:3).

Dear God, please help me to always make plans, get up and be obedient to Your commands (see Haggai 1:8).

Heavenly Father, thank You for the victory I have in You. My joy is great because of You (see Psalm 21:1).

Dear Lord, I know that unless You are the one who builds my house, all my labor is in vain. Thank You for being the master builder of my life (see Psalm 127:1).

GROUP PRAYER REQUESTS   TODAY'S DATE:_____

NAME	REQUEST	RESULTS

TWO KINDS OF WISDOM

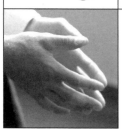

MEMORY VERSE

Who is wise and understanding among you?
Let him show it by his good life, by deeds done
in the humility that comes from wisdom
James 3:13

The apostle Paul's focus in life was to be like Christ. He admitted that he was not perfect, but that each day he pressed on to become more like Christ (see Philippians 3:12). According to Philippians 3:17-21, Paul wanted the people of Philippi to do the same. We, too, should be striving for more Christlikeness in our daily lives. We are not perfect yet, but when Christ returns we will be made perfect. Because of what Jesus did on the cross, His death for our sins guarantees that one day we will be completely perfect. In the meantime, we should continue to grow and mature spiritually, learning to make wise choices, using the heavenly wisdom we have available and distinguishing that wisdom from the earthly wisdom of this world.

In this week's study, we will examine the two kinds of wisdom that James, the brother of Jesus, wrote about in his letter to the Christians.

DAY 1: *Earthly Wisdom*

➢ According to James 3:14-15, what are the characteristics of earthly wisdom?

➢ What is the result of earthly wisdom (v. 16)?

The type of wisdom we choose to use is evidenced by our actions. Bitter envy and selfishness are two indicators of Satan's influence in our lives. Allowing unspiritual thoughts and ideas to take hold is a sure sign that you are displaying earthly—rather than heavenly—wisdom. Disorder in your life will be the result of the unwise choices you make.

➳ We have all experienced the results of unwise choices. Describe what you have experienced as a result of an unwise choice in your own life.

➳ In John 8:44, Jesus warned us about the devil's tactics. What are they?

Not only is Satan a liar, but Jesus said he is the "father of lies" (John 8:44). When we rely on our earthly wisdom, we are helping Satan carry out his plans to thwart God's work in our lives and in the world.

➳ What does 1 Peter 5:8-9 tell us about how to defend against Satan's attacks?

God has provided everything we need to avoid the earthly wisdom influenced by Satan. If we need godly wisdom for the difficulties or the questions we face, our Lord has promised to provide it *when we ask* (see James 1:5) Not only will He give us wisdom, but also He will give it generously!

 Lord, I pray You will help me refrain from using Satan's wisdom that will hinder Your work in my life. Each time I show by my actions that I am helping Satan, please convict me and set me on the straight path. Thank You for Your wisdom which You have promised to generously provide whenever I ask.

DAY 2: Heavenly Wisdom

This week's memory verse tells us that if we consider ourselves wise, we will show it by our good life and by deeds done in *humility* that comes from wisdom. One way to measure true heavenly wisdom is to look at a person's character. Just as we identify a tree by the type of fruit it yields, so we can gauge a person's wisdom by the way he or she acts. If we claim to be wise but act foolishly, we do not have true wisdom.

➤ What are the two kinds of wisdom described in James 3:13-17?

➤ List the eight characteristics of heavenly wisdom found in verse 17.

1. _____

2. _____

3. _____

4. _____

5. _____

6. _____

7. _____

8. _____

Each of us has made unwise choices at different times. God can use those times to teach us His heavenly wisdom.

The following are examples of using heavenly wisdom in following your First Place commitments. Add your plan for using heavenly wisdom to each. (The first is an example.)

➤ What will you do when you are at a buffet meal with friends?

Quickly survey the buffet to see what is available; then carefully select those foods that fit into my eating plan. Take small portions and only take one trip through the buffet line.

➤ You have decided to eliminate rich fatty desserts from your eating plan, but family and friends surprise you with cake and ice cream on your birthday. How will you stick to your plan?

➤ You planned to go walking today because you missed yesterday's walk, and it's storming outside. How will you fulfill your plan?

➤ You are determined to drink eight glasses of water every day, and a friend suggests a day of shopping. How will you insure your success of drinking enough water?

➤ You have an extremely busy day ahead and a to-do list that is a mile long. Rather than spending your usual time in Bible study and prayer, you'll skip it—just this once—say a quick prayer and get on with the day's activities. How can you keep your commitment to Bible study and prayer?

It is easier to choose earthly wisdom when faced with these kinds of choices. Heavenly wisdom requires using the knowledge God provides and making right choices. You are in training to think like Christ and become more like Him every day until He returns. Heavenly wisdom will enable you to stay on the path and make wise choices in all areas of your life.

 Dear God, I need Your heavenly wisdom in so many areas of my life. I want to take the easy path and sometimes just do nothing. I know that not choosing is choosing nonetheless. Please help me as I continue my journey in First Place and wait for Your coming.

DAY 3: *The Good Life*

As we seek wisdom for our lives, we have biblical models to use as examples. There are many ways to determine if someone has wisdom. A truly wise person puts God first, turning to Him for answers and direction. Wise people trust in the Lord when circumstances look the worst. They do what is right regardless of the consequences to themselves. They are teachable, they listen, and they give good advice. When faced with temptation, they will turn from evil. They know right from wrong, and they respect and fear God. They are genuine, loyal and kind.

➤ There are many biblical role models who practiced wisdom when faced with difficult choices. We can see their role and how they acted out their wisdom. Read about the following people and write how they showed wisdom:

- Abigail, the wise wife—1 Samuel 25:2-32

- Daniel, the wise counselor—Daniel 5:1-12,16-18

- Joseph, the wise leader—Acts 7:9-14

- Moses, the wise leader—Acts 7:30-41

➤ Write the benefits of heavenly wisdom found in each of the following Scripture passages:

- Proverbs 3:5-6

- Proverbs 3:7-8

Heavenly wisdom can be developed over time and brings with it a satisfying life, favor with God and people, health and vitality, protection and peace. It is also its own reward. We can be thankful for biblical models of heavenly wisdom and strive to practice wisdom in our own lives.

Gracious Lord, I desire to have Your heavenly wisdom. Please help me discern between it and the earthly wisdom that leads to destruction. Make me quick to recognize the good examples You have set before me, both from Your Word and through the leadership You provide.

DAY 4: *Humility*

According to Philippians 2:3, we are urged to "in humility consider others better than yourselves." But how do we show true humility without becoming prideful about our humility (see Proverbs 3:34; 1 Peter 5:5)? One common mistake people make in an attempt to *act* humble is to belittle themselves. When we demean ourselves and trample over our own worthiness, we are not showing humility—in fact, our actions might be disrespectful to our God and creator. God deems us so valuable and of such great worth that He sent His Son to die for our sins (see John 3:16). Who are we to say that the value our Creator places on us is wrong?

➤ How would you define humility?

God gives us wisdom, and as we practice humility we put ourselves in a position to be used by God for His purposes. How do we know what true humility looks like? We have the perfect model of the humble servant: Jesus Christ, our Savior.

➤ What does Philippians 2:5-8 teach us about the humility of Christ?

Jesus gave us a vivid picture of humility when He washed the feet of His disciples the night before He was crucified. Can you imagine our Savior washing your dirty feet? Read the account in John 13:1-17.

≫ How does the picture of Jesus washing your dirty feet help you to understand what true humility is? What impact does His humble act have on you?

As you lose weight and become physically healthier others will take notice. This may give you the opportunity to practice humility.

≫ If someone comments on how terrific you look and how well you have done, how can you respond in humility?

Giving God the glory for the victory you experience in First Place is one way to put Him first and live humbly. True humility does not mean putting ourselves down; it means exalting Christ above ourselves. We know that we are sinners, saved by grace. That fact alone tells us we are of great worth in God's kingdom.

O Lord, my God, I only have to look at the heavens, the moon and stars to know how majestic You are. You created me and gave me great value. I stand humbly before You, Lord, praising Your wonderful name. Help me to emulate the true humility of Your Son, my Savior.

DAY 5: *Wise Choices*

God's wisdom is there for the asking, but we must ask! If we need heavenly wisdom, all we need to do is reach out for what is readily available to us.

≫ Summarize Proverbs 9:1-6.

This proverb gives a vivid picture of the bounty of heavenly wisdom. When we make wise choices, we will be blessed.

➤ How is folly (earthly wisdom) described in Proverbs 9:13-18?

➤ Does that make foolish choices desirable?

➤ What would be wise/healthy choices to replace the following choices that you might be faced with?

Foolish Choices	Wise Alternatives
Buying a jumbo-size burger, fries and drink combo	
Watching TV for four hours every evening	
Buying a huge bag of potato chips "for the kids"	
Listening to talk radio on the way to work or to run errands	
Hitting the snooze button just one more time	

A good strategy to follow as you work to make healthy/wise choices is learning to recognize situations in which you might be faced with decisions and deciding ahead of time what the wise alternatives would be.

➤ Which type of wisdom will you choose and how will that affect your life this week?

God in heaven, I choose Your way, Your heavenly wisdom. You know best what I need and how You want to use me in Your plan for Your kingdom. I lack the understanding necessary to always make the right choice. Help me to seek Your will daily and follow the direction You provide in Your Word.

DAY 6: *Reflections*

In this week's study, you have discovered two kinds of wisdom: heavenly wisdom and earthly wisdom. You have learned the characteristics of both and which one you should rely on. It is important to remember that making wise choices is an action that may not always come easily and may not be done consistently. We have to unlearn old habits and ideas before new ones can take their place, and this process takes time.

Biblical examples show that while God's people were wise in some areas, they often made foolish choices. Don't beat yourself up when you make a choice that turns out to be poor. Through God's mercy and love, spiritual growth can come from making a wrong choice (see Romans 8:28). The examples we find in God's Word clearly show our great need for God's guidance.

Lord, help me to make wise choices. I ask for Your wisdom to guide me. Thank You that You have promised to give Your wisdom generously (see James 1:5).

Heavenly Father, guide me to choose what is right and just because that is more acceptable to You than sacrifice (see Proverbs 21:3).

Help me, Lord, to hear Your words of knowledge and apply my heart to Your instruction (see Proverbs 23:12).

DAY 7: *Reflections*

Developing heavenly wisdom takes time. God wants to teach us His way and help us acquire the characteristics of His wisdom. Those who would brag about being good and unselfish and yet harbor envy and bitterness exhibit earthly wisdom (see James 3:14-15). God wants to take us out of that, teaching us to leave behind the earthly things and to walk in His wisdom.

God also wants us to employ heavenly wisdom one choice at a time. By seeking His wisdom, sharing with your First Place group and following wise counsel, you are more likely to make wise choices, each choice empowering and strengthening you toward repeating the action. Those times when earthly wisdom wins out are opportunities to gain understanding, prompting you to not repeat that action.

Reading and memorizing God's Word are the best ways to gain godly wisdom. When you have His wisdom readily on your tongue or in your mind, it will be much easier to withstand Satan's deceptions. Every week you are provided a memory verse to learn that applies to the week's lesson. As you complete the Bible study each week, more verses are brought to your attention. One way to add to your list of memorized verses is to jot down a few verses from your study each week and begin to store up even more of God's wisdom in your heart to prepare you in times of temptation or difficulty (see Psalm 119:11).

Lord God, I want to grow in Your wisdom and knowledge (see 2 Peter 3:18). Help me to learn from my mistakes.

Father, help me hold my tongue and not be boastful about what I do. May I boast only in what You have done (see Galatians 6:14).

Heavenly Father, my desire is to serve You in humility, always putting others above myself (see Philippians 2:3).

Lord, I want to be wise and understanding. Let me show You wisdom in my life, by deeds done in the humility that comes from wisdom (see James 3:13).

GROUP PRAYER REQUESTS   TODAY'S DATE:_____

NAME	REQUEST	RESULTS

THE RIGHT OR THE WRONG HELP

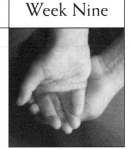

MEMORY VERSE
Some trust in chariots and some in horses,
but we trust in the name of the LORD our God.
Psalm 20:7

You may have tried what seems like every diet ever to come out, including powders and pills—perhaps even a drastic surgery. We all tend to think of weight issues as being only physical ones and fall into the trap of believing that the answers depend on our own resources, fads and quick fixes. In this week's study, we will examine two types of help available to us.

DAY 1: *Running to Egypt*

Throughout history, wars have been fought and won by nations whose weapons were superior. However, these victories are only temporary as stronger nations are continually emerging with larger and more powerful firearms. God alone has the power to preserve us; He wants us to trust in Him and come to Him for help, knowing only He can deliver us from the enemy. When we call upon almighty God for help, we are saying, "I am placing my trust in You, God, not in the weapons or ways of man."

➤ What does Isaiah 31:1 say about relying on the aid of earthly powers to save us?

In this verse, we see that Judah was trusting in man's power rather than God's almighty power. Are we doing the same if we turn to fad diets to take care of our weight problems or the latest self-help guru to help us with our out-of-control lives? That is going to Egypt for help and God says, "Woe to those who go down to Egypt for help" (Isaiah 31:1).

Name some of the places you have gone to for help or things you have done in trying to lose weight or make other lifestyle changes.

➤ According to Psalm 20:7-8, what happens to those who trust in anyone or anything except God?

➤ What happens to those who trust in God?

If we ask God to help us lose the weight or overcome a bad habit, then we will have to give up our unhealthy lifestyle choices. We may need to spend some time in repentance. The Israelites were resisting God's call for repentance (see Isaiah 31:6). They ran instead to Egypt for help. Are you resisting God's help because He requires repentance—a complete turnaround—and you don't want to make the changes you know are necessary?

➤ What are some of the things you may have to give up and repent of as you ask for God's help in your journey to a healthy, well-balanced life?

➤ Are you willing to pay the price of seeking God's help?

☐ Yes   ☐ No

❧ According to Jeremiah 29:11, what does God want to do?

❧ What is the rest of the promise, and what is our part in the promise found in verses 12 and 13?

When we pray to God, He is always listening. When we seek Him, we will find Him. We do not need to run to Egypt—other fad diets or programs—for help. Our help is right here for the asking.

 All-powerful God, You hold me in Your hand and preserve me. Thank You, Lord, for Your strength and power. I want to trust in You and always come to You for the help I need. I confess that in the past, I've gone to Egypt for help, only to be left with failure. I should have trusted You because You will never fail me. Help me always to look to You for victory.

DAY 2: *Horses and Chariots*

Look once again at Isaiah 31:1. Sturdy chariots pulled by swift horses had a decided advantage over the ordinary foot soldier. They could run farther and faster than a person on foot. However, chariots and horses have their limit; they wear out or break down. As we face the battle of trying to lose weight and/or get fit, we might believe that we need the chariots and horses of food substitutes, pills or other aids to carry us to instant victory in the battle.

❧ Name things that you rely on (besides depending on God) to help you lose weight or stop a bad habit.

For many people, weight or health problems might be the result of inner struggles over past hurts, anger, sin, rejection or bitterness. When these are unresolved, depression and other problems develop. When inner struggles result in physical problems, we can be so anxious to end the physical problem instantly that we hop on a moving chariot pulled by swift horses and head off to Egypt for help.

➤ What is something that might be an underlying cause of your weight or other physical problems?

➤ Have you trusted God with your inner struggles? Why or why not?

➤ How have you seen progress in this area since you have been in First Place?

➤ Explain Psalm 33:16-22 in your own words.

➤ What hope do you find in Psalm 33?

Perhaps you are struggling with rejection, victimization, anger or loneliness. It might be jealousy, regret or fear that has caused years of conflict in your life. Whatever your struggle may be, you can trust God to heal you. He works on the inside first so that the weight loss may come later. Trust God, even when you do not see results. He will never abandon you in the battle. The victory will be yours.

 Heavenly Father, I am guilty of climbing aboard chariots and have been swiftly carried away to Egypt for help. I have trusted in them when I should have placed my trust in You. Forgive me, Lord, and help me to remember that You are the victor because of Your awesome power.

DAY 3: *The Horsemen's Fleeting Strength*

➤ What does Isaiah 31:3 say about the Egyptians and their horses?

➤ What will happen to those they would help?

The horsemen's limited strength could not compare to God's power. When the Lord decides to stretch out His hand against anyone in opposition to Him, they and those they are trying to help will come crashing down together.

In First Place you made a commitment to God, not to a fad program. You learn to rely on Him to help you make lifestyle changes. It is God's strength that gets you through the struggle, and His power that changes you from the inside out.

➤ How has God been working in your life during this session of First Place?

In joining First Place, you have made a wise choice—seeking God's help. Although you may have not reached your goal yet, be assured that God is still working and will continue His work in you.

➣ Have you hit an obstacle in your First Place journey? Describe it.

Remember that God has the power to help you overcome any obstacle. Ask Him for His wisdom to make wise choices and continue on to victory.

 King of kings, You are all-powerful. You can provide the strength and victory I need in my journey to a healthier lifestyle. Help me to overcome the obstacles I am facing and to trust only in Your strength.

DAY 4: *Look to the Holy One*

The Lord wants to work in your life, helping and guiding you. When He hears your cry, He graciously, with compassion, answers the need in your life.

➣ Read Isaiah 30:18-21 and write down what this passage means to you.

In spite of the many times we jump aboard a chariot, God longs to be gracious and compassionate to us. Pause here and thank God for His graciousness and compassion toward you.

God allows hard times in your life, but He promises to go through them with you. He demands a lot from you, just as you demand much from those close to you. Why? Because He loves you. Just as you want to be there for your loved ones when necessary, God promises to be there for you.

Consider a recent difficult experience you went through. Be specific in describing the details as you explore the situation and its effect on your life.

≫ What was the difficult situation?

≫ How did God answer?

≫ Did He ask you to do something about the situation? Did you do it? Why or why not?

≫ What was the result?

As you look to God for help, know that He hears your plea and He will answer. The answer may not always come in the way you expect, but God *will* answer. He may ask you to take some action to cooperate with Him in bringing about a solution. As you take a step of faith, taking the action He directs, God will stand and fight your battle. Remember that your heavenly Father will not push His way into your life; He waits to be asked (see Revelation 3:20).

≫ What is one area in your life where you specifically need God's help in attaining victory?

O Lord, my God, I cry out to You for help with this area of my life that I have been unsuccessful in gaining victory. I look only to You; please hear my prayer and answer me. I will do whatever You say, Lord, keeping my eyes on You, waiting for Your answer.

DAY 5: *Seek God's Help*

No matter where you are in your journey to achieve a healthy body, whether you are well on your way to meeting your weight-loss goal, have just begun to take the steps toward your goal or anywhere in between, God will meet you there.

Sometimes, in the midst of our troubles and distress, it is difficult to see how God is working in a given situation. We may have to experience distress and difficulty in order to understand how gracious and merciful God is. He wants to reach down and gather you close because He loves you. He will never harm or abandon you; He is waiting for you now to cry out for His help and to earnestly seek Him.

➤ According to Deuteronomy 4:29-31, how do you seek God?

➤ Are you ready to do that? Explain your answer.

➤ Have you ever felt abandoned by someone? If so, by whom and why?

When you joined First Place, you made a commitment to God and asked Him to help you with your weight problem. He has never abandoned or given up on you, even if you may have stopped making the right choices or you gave up waiting for God to take off the weight for you. God has been busy working on the inside. He will not do for you what He wants you to do. Your commitment or covenant with God means He does His part and you do yours.

➤ In Psalm 139:23-24, what does David ask God to do? Can you honestly pray that prayer?

➤ According to Psalm 44:20-21, how much does God know about us?

➤ According to Psalm 94:11, what does God know about the thoughts of man?

➤ What will God discover when He looks into your heart?

Precious Lord, God of heaven and Earth, search my heart and show me what I need to see in my life. Only You know my deepest thoughts, those that are hidden even from me. I need Your help, Lord, and I seek You with all my heart and soul.

DAY 6: *Reflections*

In what do you place your trust? Think back and consider the various times of difficulty you have encountered. Where did you turn for help in trying to solve those problems? It is important to look at the past as a way to evaluate your pattern of trust placement.

When you consistently seek the world's solutions to your problems, you are not placing your trust in God. Many people follow fads such as the newest protein diet or diving into the hottest new project. These people think that because so many others are doing it, it must be the answer. This week's memory verse cautions you about putting your trust in things or people rather than in God.

How often have you kept inner struggles hidden until they became so unbearable you tried to get rid of them any way you could? You will soon discover that riding on a chariot pulled by swift horses may get you somewhere faster, but where it takes you may not be where you wanted to go. God points you to where you will find help—Him.

 Father, You are my source of help in times of trouble. Remind me to always run to You (see Psalm 46:1).

Father God, no matter what difficulties come into my life, I know I don't need to be afraid because I have You (see Isaiah 41:10).

DAY 7: *Reflections*

In this week's study, you have seen but a glimpse of God's mighty power. All of the armies of the world cannot outperform, outfight or subdue an enemy like God can. Even with humankind's knowledge, technological skills and powerful energy sources, we cannot begin to touch the unfathomable power of almighty God.

➻ Read and then summarize each of the following verses that examine God's power:

- 1 Chronicles 29:11

- Psalm 68:35

- Isaiah 40:10

- Romans 1:16

- Ephesians 1:19-20

Think about how God's power in your life has changed you. Sometimes we overlook what God has done in our lives and instead focus on all that still needs doing. Life is a journey, and if we are not careful, we will miss the beauty God has provided along the roads we travel on the way to reaching our goals. Choosing to ask God for help will make your road easier to travel, regardless of the goal you are reaching for.

 Almighty God, I praise You. You are an awesome God who gives strength to His people. You are a sovereign Lord who comes with power, providing salvation for everyone who believes. You raised Jesus from the dead and give eternal life to anyone who calls upon His name. I praise You, Lord.

Some trust in chariots and some in horses, but I will trust in the name of the Lord, my God (see Psalm 20:7).

GROUP PRAYER REQUESTS   TODAY'S DATE:_____

NAME	REQUEST	RESULTS

THE MOST IMPORTANT CHOICE

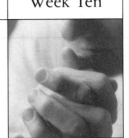

MEMORY VERSE

For God so loved the world that he gave his one and only Son, that whoever believes in him shall not perish but have eternal life.

John 3:16

As you begin the last week in this study about making wise choices, you come now to making the most important choice of all—choosing to accept Jesus Christ as your personal Lord and Savior. Perhaps you made this wise choice long ago or maybe even recently. But if you haven't, this final study will help you reexamine where you stand spiritually and guide you toward making the ultimate wise choice.

If you are already a Christian, this study will help you learn more about sharing your faith and leading others to know Jesus. This week's study will also be an opportunity to bathe in the reality of God's love for you and to evaluate where you are in your walk with the Lord, setting new goals toward reaching maturity.

DAY 1: *God Loves You So Much*

Can you imagine someone you know laying down his or her life for you? Even if your parent, spouse or friend would be willing to lay down his or her life, that act would not provide you forgiveness of sin and eternal life in heaven with God. Read about the One who has already done that in 1 John 4:9-10.

➽ Check the box that indicates whether you agree or disagree with each of the following statements:

I have committed sins.	☐ Agree	☐ Disagree
I believe God loves me.	☐ Agree	☐ Disagree
I know I am going to heaven.	☐ Agree	☐ Disagree

➤ Have you ever felt unloved or unlovable because of your physical appearance?

➤ Is there anything that you have ever done that makes you feel that you are not deserving of God's love?

God loves you regardless of what you weigh or anything you have done wrong. His actions speak loudly of His love.

➤ Read Romans 5:8 and comment on the significance of this act of love.

Jesus Christ, God's only Son, died on the cross to pay for our sins so that you could be with Him in heaven for eternity.

 Heavenly Father, thank You for sending Your Son, Jesus Christ, to pay for my sins. I cannot even imagine how painful it must have been for You to see the sins of the world—including mine—and know that the only payment for them would be for Your only Son to go to the cross. Forgive me. I receive the forgiveness You so graciously and mercifully give.

DAY 2: *He Gave His Only Son*

Romans 3:23 clearly states, "for all have sinned and fall short of the glory of God." Every one of us, by virtue of the fact that we are born into this world, has sinned. Why did Jesus have to suffer and die on the cross for our sins?

➤ According to Romans 5:12, through whom did sin enter the world? (See also Genesis 3.)

➤ What is the result of sin?

Sin separates us from God. Therefore, to live eternally in heaven, we must be free from sin. In Old Testament times, God provided a way for the forgiveness of sins through the temple sacrifices.

⟫ Hebrews 9:22 tells us what is required for sin to be forgiven. What is it?

⟫ According to Hebrews 9:26-28a, what is now the only acceptable sacrifice for sin?

⟫ In His mercy and love for us, His creation, God gave up His only Son. How does it make you feel to know that God did this for you?

⟫ Do you have difficulty forgiving yourself for past sins? Are there sins that you feel God cannot forgive or forget? Explain.

Read Romans 4:7-8. Once you have accepted Him as Savior, the Lord will never count your sin against you. When you confess your sin to God, He forgives and forgets.

⟫ Today, confess your sin to God and receive His forgiveness. Tell Him your concerns about forgiving yourself. He is a loving and merciful God and waits for you to call upon Him.

Heavenly Father, I know I have sinned and fallen short of Your glory. Please forgive my sins—past, present and future. Help me to know Your mercy and love and to be able to forgive myself. Thank You for loving me and for sending Your only Son, Jesus Christ, to provide eternal life for me.

DAY 3: *If You Believe in Him*

Admitting you are a sinner is the first step to becoming a child of God. Whether you did that yesterday or 30 years ago, you made a wise choice. The next step is to believe in Jesus Christ. God predetermined that whoever believes in Him will have eternal life.

≫ In John 3:36, what does it say you must do to have eternal life?

≫ What will happen if you reject Jesus Christ?

Again, it comes down to choosing between life and death. If you want life, choose God's Son, Jesus Christ, as your Savior. If you reject Him, you are choosing death.

Having intellectual knowledge about Jesus is not the same as knowing and trusting in Jesus Christ for salvation. Many have heard about Him but have chosen to shut Him out of their lives. Others believe that He was a great teacher who lived long ago, but they do not recognize Him as God's Son, resurrected from the dead. Even Satan and his demons know who Christ is, but that does not change their actions. True belief is demonstrated in your actions.

≫ What do you believe about Jesus Christ?

≫ How is your belief in Jesus demonstrated in your actions?

Lord Jesus Christ, I do believe that You are God's Son, who went to the cross for me to pay for my sins. I am choosing to believe in You, and I know Your Word says that if I do, I will have eternal life in heaven with You. Thank You for being my Savior.

DAY 4: *You Shall Not Perish*

God's desire is for everyone to have eternal life. He wants it so much that He very patiently waits for you to make the right choice. He promises that *whoever* comes to Him will not perish. That is a guarantee! Making wise choices involves being able to understand the consequences of wrong ones and the benefits of wise ones. A guarantee of eternal life is proof that choosing to accept Jesus Christ as your Savior is the wise choice.

➤ After reading 2 Peter 3:9, fill in the missing words.

The Lord . . . is _____ with you, not

wanting anyone to _____, but every-

one to come to _____.

Throughout God's Word, wherever He gives us a choice between life and death, we are always encouraged to choose life. He has given us understanding so that we can make a wise choice (see 1 John 5:20).

➤ What does God want you to choose?

➤ Look up the word "perish" in the dictionary and then write what it means in your own words.

Disobedience to God can result in the deterioration of our spiritual, physical, mental and emotional health, which can lead to a premature death.

≫ List some areas of disobedience in your life.

Ask God's forgiveness for the disobedience, thanking Him for His mercy and compassion.

 Precious Lord, I know I have been disobedient in certain areas of my life. I want to live and serve You as long as possible and I need Your help in changing my life, turning it around so that it honors You. Please help me do that. Thank You for Your mercy and compassion, for loving me and providing the way to eternal life.

DAY 5: *Have Eternal Life*

God's Word repeatedly provides us with assurance that whoever believes in Jesus Christ for salvation has eternal life. God does not lie; He keeps His promises. The more you read His Word, the more you will get to know Him. The Bible is God's love letter to you, showing you who He is and His purpose in your life. The most important choice you will ever make in your lifetime is whether or not you want Jesus Christ to be your Lord and Savior. When you accept Him as your Savior, you will immediately have eternal life with Him here and in heaven. If you don't, you will perish and spend eternity in hell.

≫ Read the following Scriptures and then write what each says about eternal life:

- John 3:15

- John 3:36

- John 5:24

- Romans 6:23

- 1 Timothy 1:16

- 1 John 5:11-12

- 1 John 5:13

You can know for sure that if you died today you would go to heaven and spend eternity with God. It is as simple as ABC.

A Admit to God that you are a sinner.
B Believe and receive Jesus Christ as God's Son and your Savior, accepting God's forgiveness of sin.
C Commit your life to Jesus Christ.

➤ If you have never asked Jesus to be your Savior, pray a prayer similar to the following:

Heavenly Father, I know I have sinned, and I need Your forgiveness. Thank You for sending Your Son to pay the price for my sin. I believe in Jesus Christ, that He died on the cross so I can have eternal life. By faith, I am accepting Jesus as my Savior. I want Him to reside in my heart and be Lord of my life. Thank You for loving me unconditionally and helping me make the most important choice of all. Amen.

Welcome into the family of God. Now, call your First Place leader and share your good news. You have just made the most important choice of your life, and your leader will want to help you as you begin your journey toward spiritual maturity.

If you have accepted Jesus as your Savior and Lord, evaluate the state of your relationship with Him. Are you continuing to grow toward spiritual maturity, or has your walk with God been slowed to a snail's pace or even a standstill? What is missing in your relationship with Him? Spend some time in prayer, talking to God. Then sit down with your journal, listen to what He tells you and write it down.

DAY 6: *Reflections*

The final week of this study on making wise choices brings us back around to the beginning. During the first week, you learned about choosing between life and death and that God urges us to choose life. We have come full circle as we conclude the study with Jesus telling us the same thing in John 3:16. He told us how much God loves us, how much He gave up for us and how we will benefit from making the right choice.

God is concerned with everything you do, everything that bothers you and everything that affects you. Most of all, He is concerned about your soul. God's desire is that you spend eternity with Him. He wants the best for you.

For several weeks now, we have studied the importance of making wise choices. We have discussed the benefits of making wise choices and the consequences of making unwise choices. If you have not yet made the decision to trust God with your soul, won't you do that today?

Study Romans 10:9-10. If you have accepted Jesus Christ as Savior—whether years ago or today—you must not be ashamed to confess your faith to others. If you have never done so, share your faith story with another person. Read "Sharing Your Faith" on pages 29-30 in the *First Place Member's Guide* if you have never done this before. If you have made the ultimate wise choice to follow Jesus just in the last day or so, call your First Place leader or another group member and share your good news.

 Precious Savior and Lord, thank You so much for Your unfathomable gift of eternal life. Thank You too for the gift of Your Holy Spirit now living in me and who will teach me about You (see John 14:16,26).

Help me, O God, to walk in a manner worthy of my calling as a believer in You (see Ephesians 4:1).

Strengthen me, Lord, to confess with my mouth, "Jesus is Lord" (see Romans 10:9). Help me to tell others of Your gift of eternal life through Jesus Christ.

DAY 7: *Reflections*

Have you been a child of God many years or just a few days? Perhaps you accepted Jesus Christ when you were young but strayed over the years. Or perhaps you made this choice after becoming an adult but have grown weary from dealing with life's struggles. Becoming a Christian guarantees you that you will enter heaven and spend eternity with God. It doesn't, however, guarantee a stress-free, easy life while you are on Earth. So you may be wondering, *What is the purpose of all this?*

The benefits of your salvation began the moment you made the choice of accepting Jesus Christ as your Savior. At that moment, Jesus sent the Holy Spirit to reside in your heart (see John 16:7). When you ask the Holy Spirit for help, you no longer struggle alone. His power, encouragement, wisdom and comfort will see you through every trial you face.

Even if you have not experienced total victory this session, you can trust God and know that He is steadily at work in you. His desire is that you become all that He meant you to be. God will not give up on you. You must not give up on Him. Remember that success is all about making wise, godly choices.

If you have already made the wise choice of becoming a child of God, you may want to recommit your life to Him. Perhaps you are not as active in sharing your faith with others as you would like. Maybe you wish your prayer life were more dynamic. Ask God to give you a burden for lost sinners and a passion for studying His Word. There are many who will perish unless Christians reach out and share the gospel of Jesus Christ.

Congratulations on making the wisest choice of your life. Please tell someone about the choice you have made. Whether it was becoming a new Christian or recommitting your life to Him, it was a wise choice and one that should be shared. Tell your leader, your pastor or a friend. Let someone rejoice with you just as God is rejoicing right now.

 Holy Father God, thank You for the unspeakable gift of Your precious Son, Jesus, for my eternal life (see John 3:16). There is no greater gift that can be given than Your life for me, a sinner. Praise Your holy name!

GROUP PRAYER REQUESTS TODAY'S DATE:_____

NAME	REQUEST	RESULTS

BECOMING A
TOTAL PERSON

And Jesus grew in wisdom and stature, and in favor with God and men.
Luke 2:52

Even Christians can become frustrated with life, missing the love, joy, peace and fulfillment that should be dominant in their lives. Believers can be lonely and feeling on the verge of hopelessness. Some may suffer from poor health; others may feel that depression is just a way of life. Many may ask, "Is this the full life that Jesus promised us in John's Gospel?" (see John 10:10). Christians who fit any of these descriptions are not experiencing what it means to be a total person.

On a scale of 1 to 10, with 1 experiencing hopelessness and 10 experiencing abundant life, where do you fit in? Place an X on the following scale where you would assess your life right now:

1	2	3	4	5	6	7	8	9	10

Hopelessness   Abundant Life

"What exactly *is* a total person?" you might ask. The answer is probably different than what you expect. First, here is what being a total person *isn't*: (1) one who is morally perfect; (2) one who is spiritually perfect; (3) one who experiences a state of perpetual bliss and contentment; (4) one who expects to receive unconditional love or acceptance from others.

It may surprise you, but there is one more thing a total person is not: completely fulfilled. A God-inspired discontent within us keeps us continually seeking, searching and growing toward the ultimate that is complete union with God and His will. That perfect union will be realized in a way that we cannot comprehend until it is experienced when we reach the place Jesus has prepared for us (see John 14:3). Therefore, the wholeness we attain here on Earth will not be constant or complete, but we can experience in part what we will completely attain when we go to heaven.

Simply stated, being a total person implies one who has a healthy mind, body and spirit and also has healthy relationships and attitudes. A total person is one who lives in conformity with God's will and standards and is happy to do so, acquiring patience within and toward others. The total person has learned to build up a tolerance for the frustrations and anxieties that besiege every individual. The total person learns to deal with disappointment, futility, confusion and occasional failure in healthy, constructive ways.

Growth toward becoming a total person involves learning to give, whether it be love, money, encouragement or time. When we learn to give, we soon discover that the very act of giving is therapeutic to our own personalities and our interpersonal relationships. It helps speed our growth toward maturity and wholeness. Jesus realized this important segment of our personality by giving us this directive: "I tell you the truth, whatever you did for one of the least of these brothers of mine, you did for me" (Matthew 25:40). God's Word also states "It is more blessed to give than to receive" (Acts 20:35).

➤ How can you develop a giving attitude? Make a list of people that you can give to and then how you will give them love, money, encouragement or time. (For example, you might write "I will give my time to Sarah by taking her out to lunch this week.")

- I will give love to _____
  by _____.

- I will give my resources to _____
  by _____.

- I will give encouragement to _____
  by _____.

- I will give my time to _____
  by _____.

In our desire to develop into a total person, we need to focus our attention on Jesus. We can use His perfect example to see how we should live our lives. Luke 2:52 gives us some revealing hints about the ways in which Jesus developed in four major areas in His life. "And Jesus grew in wisdom and stature, and in favor with God and men."

Jesus developed mentally (wisdom), physically (stature), spiritually (in favor with God) and emotionally (in favor with men).

We all have mental, physical, spiritual and emotional needs, so we must continuously grow and develop in each of these areas. If we neglect one of these areas, it will experience decay which in turn will affect other dimensions of our person. We are told in 1 Corinthians 12:26, "If one part suffers, every part suffers with it; if one part is honored, every part rejoices with it." Many Christians may be healthy in their spiritual and emotional needs but unhealthy in their mental and physical selves. The confusions and frustrations caused from being unhealthy in these areas will affect the spiritual and emotional dimensions. We must learn to develop our health in all four areas so that we can develop into the total person, just as our Savior did.

 Lord, cause me to grow in all four areas—spiritually, emotionally, mentally and physically. Restore to me the joy that Your salvation brings and give me a willing spirit to sustain me (see Psalm 51:12).

MENTAL DEVELOPMENT

And Jesus grew in wisdom.

Luke 2:52

During His life, Jesus demonstrated scholarly growth and development. In Luke 2:47 we learn how the young Jesus amazed the scholarly priests with His knowledge of Scripture. Was this because Jesus was born with this knowledge? No. Although Jesus is the Son of God, He was sent to this earth as an infant. He had to grow, learn and develop just as all of us have to do. He spent many, many hours in concentrated study of the Scriptures, improving His knowledge of God's Word, as did all Jewish boys of His day.

Many Christians fail to cultivate their mental faculties. Watching soap operas on TV, reading romance novels and magazines, and attending movies that portray violence and sex are activities that are not going to contribute significantly to positive mental growth.

One rule that must be understood for effective learning is *the overload principle*. This principle is basic in developing all four areas—mental, physical, spiritual and emotional—in your life. To learn effectively, you must consistently place a positive overload on your mental capabilities. Read educational books, watch TV programs that contribute to your knowledge and attend lectures or seminars that can broaden your education.

An extremely important way to improve your mental capacity is through Scripture memorization. When you consistently hide God's Word in your heart you will replace the lies in your mind with the truth of God. Ask God to show you Scriptures (in addition to your First Place Bible study verses) to meditate on and memorize. Listen for these verses in sermons, Bible classes or in conversations with others.

After asking God to bring specific Scriptures to mind, make a list of those Scripture passages you want to start memorizing. Add to the list as you read and study God's Word.

Many times fear, feelings of inadequacy or even laziness can keep us from taking a step out of our mundane lives and into new ventures.

However, the Scriptures teach us that fear does not come from God; rather, power, love and discipline do (see 2 Timothy 1:7). Seek God's power and list some topics that you would like to learn more about or educational opportunities you may like to pursue.

≫ Things I would like to learn more about

≫ Classes, seminars, or studies I would like to attend

God has created in you a tremendous potential for mental development. Do not allow this immeasurable potential to go stagnant. Do not be afraid or too lazy to learn about new areas of life. Develop your God-given potential by consistently overloading your mind with positive educational thoughts. Fulfilling each of the First Place commitments is a positive step forward in increasing your knowledge. The physical commitments increase your knowledge of nutritional fitness. The spiritual commitments increase your knowledge of God, His way and your personal relationship with Him.

EMOTIONAL DEVELOPMENT

And Jesus grew . . . in favor with men.
Luke 2:52

The Bible tells us that Jesus developed His emotional needs by attending weddings, religious functions and on many occasions, dining with friends. Our emotional needs can be satisfied with positive interpersonal relationships with one another.

Before we can establish healthy relationships with others, we must first learn to love ourselves. This doesn't mean loving yourself in a selfish manner; this is not love, it is self-centeredness. Loving yourself in a godly manner means liking yourself the way you are, the way you feel, the way you think and the way you behave. If you don't like yourself in these areas, you will not be able to love others, because they will also conflict with you in these areas. For example, a person who is overweight might not like his or her appearance. This person's feelings about the way he or she looks will cause emotional conflicts and can cause a resentment toward others who are more physically fit. Obviously, this resentment would cause a loss in the ability to be a witness for Christ. Jesus understood this when He gave the directive, "Love your neighbor as yourself" (Matthew 22:39).

➤ Make a list of your strengths, gifts and abilities.

Thank God for each item on your list and pray Psalm 139:14 over your life.

Lord, I am fearfully and wonderfully made. Wonderful are Your works and my soul knows it very well!

After you learn to love yourself, the second thing you must do is to learn how to love others—even the unlovely and unlovable. We all know that God loves us, regardless of how unlovable we might be. During the time when Jesus walked the earth as a man, He loved every type of person as well—the rich, the poor, the intellectual, the simpleminded, His friends and His enemies. His commands are: "Love your neighbor as yourself" (Matthew 22:39), and "Love your enemies and pray for those who persecute you" (Matthew 5:44).

Always be willing to welcome new friends. Seek out people with varied interests, backgrounds and cultures. Learn and share ideas with these newfound friends. This giving and receiving from the new interpersonal relationships will enhance your emotional well-being and will help you on your journey toward becoming a total person.

Do you have any unlovable people in your life? Have you attempted to love them? If not, ask God to develop a love for them in your heart, and as you pray seek out opportunities to include those people in your life. Here are just a few ideas for reaching out to others.

- Sit next to someone you do not know at the next worship service, PTA meeting or business meeting, and introduce yourself.
- Host a neighborhood get-together.
- Take a meal to a neighbor who may be ill or to a new mother in your church.

There are many ways in which you can reach out to others and develop relationships with those whom you might not have considered as potential friends in the past. Don't be afraid to use your creativity and develop your own plan—you will find your interpersonal relationships blossoming as you continue to seek out new friendships and enhance your emotional well-being.

SPIRITUAL DEVELOPMENT

And Jesus grew in . . . favor with God.
Luke 2:52

Jesus spent time developing a close relationship with His heavenly Father. His heartfelt desire to know God better is one that we should try to duplicate.

Are you aware of the resources God has provided for leading a rich and exciting life? The untapped potential lies within the grasp of each one of us, yet it can be easy to lead a mediocre, roller-coaster existence of occasional mountaintop experiences followed by slides back into the same rut—and we might conclude that this must be the normal Christian life. But thankfully, Jesus came so that believers might have life "to the full" (John 10:10). If we are willing to pay the price, God will lead us into fulfillment and adventure with Him. The following principles and guidelines can help us develop our spiritual growth.

GOD'S RESOURCES AND PERSONAL EFFORT

The purpose of growing in Christ is to reflect His character and minister to others so that they may come to know Him.

According to the Bible, Christians do not grow just by their own effort but by the actions of God's Spirit within. It is the believer's responsibility to spend time and energy fulfilling God's requirements for growth.

Frantic efforts to develop spiritual wholeness on your own or a lackadaisical leave-it-all-to-God attitude do not produce growth. Christians are called both to rely on God's resources and to respond in obedience to Him.

How can you develop reliance on God through your own efforts? First, commit to showing up to your First Place meetings. Do your Bible study on a daily basis. Make a commitment to use your First Place *Prayer Journal* daily to write out your thoughts and prayers and the ways in which God answers them. Finally, set aside a special place and time in your daily life to spend alone with God.

LIVE IN THE FULLNESS OF THE HOLY SPIRIT

All who commit their lives to Christ receive the Holy Spirit. However, many Christians still do not yield to Him or rely on the resources He brings into their lives. Through ignorance or rebellion, they miss the abundant life Christ promised.

If we are to live in the fullness of the Holy Spirit, we must confess all known sin and accept God's cleansing by faith. Confession of all known sin brings cleansing from all unrighteousness (see 1 John 1:9). This will bring a feeling of peace and freedom to your life.

Another way to live in the fullness of the Holy Spirit is to yield all areas of your life to Jesus (see Romans 12:1-2). Many Christians are afraid to totally yield their lives either because they have sins they want to retain or because they fear God will cheat them out of a really full life if they submit to Him.

We must realize that God intends what is best for us (see Jeremiah 29:11). His desire is that we spend our lives on things of everlasting value, not on impressive and attractive things of this world (see Matthew 6:33). With the help of His power, commit yourself to break from those things displeasing to Him and develop those habits and activities that honor Him.

Hebrews 12:1 tells us to "throw off everything that hinders and the sin that so easily entangles." What sin in your life is hindering you from living in the fullness of the Holy Spirit? Confess this sin to God, telling Him that you have not been obedient in this specific area. Repent and return to God's ways (see Acts 3:19). Ask God to forgive you and He will (see 1 John 1:9).

GROW IN YOUR PERSONAL KNOWLEDGE OF GOD

Start Your Day Off Right

In order to get to know God, you must spend time with Him and learn more about Him. Personal relationships demand personal time together. Even Jesus found it necessary to set aside a special time for communication with His Father (see Mark 1:35).

Our time with God before the day starts will set the tone for all we do that day. Yield to God in prayer for control and filling of your life. Express thanks and praise to Him. Begin your day praying over matters that will affect you that day.

Study God's Word

Gain a practical grasp of God's Word. An understanding of the Bible will help you develop a closer relationship with your heavenly Father. One of the major reasons many Christians do not live a fuller life is that they are ignorant of the Bible's teachings. This causes them to fall into sin. Listening, reading, studying and meditating on the Word of God are necessary for knowing Him and being obedient to His will.

Apply God's Word

Once you have studied Scripture, you must practically apply it to your life in order to develop an even greater understanding of who God is. One way to do this is to make the verses personal. For example, consider Ecclesiastes 5:5 which says, "It is better not to vow than to make a vow and not fulfill it." Determine to not make any commitment unless you intend to fulfill it. Then live out the commitment daily when asked to volunteer for a job or complete a task for someone. Finally, pray the verse into your life.

 Lord, help me to only make commitments that I can keep. Remind me, Father, to make wise decisions when opportunities to make commitments come my way (see Ecclesiastes 5:5).

USE OPPORTUNITIES TO MINISTER TO OTHERS

A key part of God's plan for our spiritual growth is service. What we receive from Him, He desires that we use to minister to others.

Find a Church Home

We can minister to others about God's grace by becoming a part of a fellowship of Christians. Through becoming a member of a church, you will not only have the opportunity to help others but you also will learn and receive encouragement from others. Having a church home provides a community that can keep you accountable and help you when extra support is needed.

Share Christ with Others

Learn to share Christ with others around you. If you yield to God and ask Him, He will use you to share the good news about Christ. Your experience in the First Place program can be a wonderful witnessing tool. When asked about how you have lost weight or why your life has changed, you can take the opportunity to share your own testimony or a special Scripture.

Do you have friends and acquaintances whom you know are not Christians? Share with these nonbelievers how prayer and Bible study have helped change your life. Invite them to the First Place Victory Celebration and then use that opportunity to invite them to participate in the next First Place study.

Utilize God's resources (His promises, His Spirit, His Word and His church) for spiritual growth. First Place is a great program that will encourage proper use of these resources and will help you as you develop into a total person.

PHYSICAL DEVELOPMENT

And Jesus grew in . . . stature.

Luke 2:52

There is evidence that Jesus once walked a distance of 120 miles in a three-day period (see Mark 5—6). It would have been impossible to walk those great distances in a short time if Jesus had not been in excellent cardiovascular condition. His daylong journeys often took Him up to 50 miles a day through rugged mountainous terrain (see Matthew 15:21,29).

In His early life Jesus was a carpenter. His work required Him to possess a great amount of strength. He did not have the luxury of power tools to aid Him. It took strength and physical endurance just to saw a board. Jesus' strength and condition was evident on the day He was crucified; only a well-conditioned man could have survived the beating and torture that preceded His crucifixion, not to mention the emotional and mental pain He was in. Then He carried the cross beam at least partway to Golgotha. It was only along the road that we see Him falter. Even though another man carried the beam the rest of the way, Jesus had to still walk up the hill to His crucifixion.

The physical potential that each person possesses can be reached only through exercise that physiologists describe as the overload principle. To gain strength or skill, an overload (whether it be a heavy weight or a long practice) must be placed on our present physical ability. The degree of overload will determine the increase in our physical ability. The smaller the overload, the smaller the increase; the larger the overload, the larger the increase.

This overload must be applied in the health-related components of physical fitness. Those areas are cardiovascular-respiratory fitness, body composition, muscular strength and endurance fitness, and flexibility fitness. To achieve total fitness, we must adopt an exercise plan that includes work (an overload on what was previously done) in all these areas.

Your exercise plan should include activities in each of the following three categories:

1. Aerobic activity
2. Flexibility or stretching
3. Strength training

Do you have an exercise plan in place? If not, start now to develop a plan that will help you to achieve total physical fitness. Use the following chart to help you get started with your fitness plan:

	AEROBIC	STRENGTH	FLEXIBILITY
MONDAY			
TUESDAY			
WEDNESDAY			
THURSDAY			
FRIDAY			
SATURDAY			
SUNDAY			

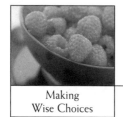

FIRST PLACE
MENU PLANS

VEGETARIAN MENU EXCHANGES

Each plan is based on approximately 1,400 calories.

Breakfast   2 breads, 1 fruit, 1 milk, 0-½ fat
(When a meat exchange is used, milk is omitted.)

Lunch   2 meat alternatives, 2 breads, 1 vegetable, 1 fruit, 1 fat

Dinner   2-3 meat alternatives, 2-3 breads, 2 vegetables, 1-2 fats

Snacks   1 meat alternative, 1 fruit, 1 milk, 1-1½ fats (or any
remaining exchanges)

For more calories, add the following to the 1,400 calorie plan.

1,600 calories   2 breads, 1 fat

1,800 calories   2 meat alternatives, 3 breads, 1 vegetable, 1 fat

2,000 calories   2 meat alternatives, 4 breads, 1 vegetable, 3 fats

2,200 calories   2 meat alternatives, 5 breads, 1 vegetable, 1 fruit, 5 fats

2,400 calories   2 meat alternatives, 6 breads, 2 vegetables, 1 fruit, 6 fats

The exchanges for these meals were calculated using the MasterCook software. It uses a database of over 6,000 food items prepared using United States Department of Agriculture (USDA) publications and information from food manufacturers. As with any nutritional program, MasterCook calculates the nutritional values of the recipes based on ingredients. Nutrition may vary due to how the food is prepared, where the food comes from, soil content, season, ripeners, processing and method of preparation. For these reasons, please use the recipes and menu plans as approximate guides. As always, consult your physician and/or a registered dietician before starting a diet program.

A Note from Chef Scott

I hope that you enjoy these new vegetarian menu selections. If you are familiar with the different vegetarian lifestyles, you will notice that these menus are not vegan (i.e., no animal products); they are ovo-lacto vegetarian (i.e., containing eggs and dairy products).

Meat Alternatives

Many menus use meat alternatives. These can be found in most major grocery stores. Look in the nutrition, freezer and produce sections— the location may vary by store. Some brands to look for are Boca, Yve's, Lightlife, Morningstar Farms and Galaxy. These products are mainly vegan but may contain some dairy products.

Soy Milk versus Dairy Milk

If you prefer to use soy milk instead of dairy milk, be sure to choose a soy milk that is *calcium fortified* and either reduced fat or nonfat. Many vegan soy cheeses are also available—compare the nutritional information to make the right choices. Whether substituting soy products for milk or cheese, be sure to make the appropriate changes in your exchange information.

About Tofu

Tofu is pretty bland, and since it has virtually no flavor of its own, it will take on the flavors of the food it is cooked with. I think you'll find the following tips useful:

- Tofu can be frozen and then grated to give your dishes a meatier texture.
- When using firm tofu in stir-fry dishes, be sure to drain and press the tofu blocks to remove excess moisture. The easiest way to do this is in the kitchen sink. Place the tofu between two heavy plates; place a weight on the top plate, making it heavy enough to force out the excess moisture within 20 to 30 minutes.

- You can keep a partial package of tofu up to one week. Simply use the amount your recipe calls for; then cover and refrigerate, replacing liquid with water each day to retain consistency.

- Use firm and extra-firm tofu for stir-frying.

- Substitute soft and silken varieties of tofu for eggs in recipes. These varieties can also be used in place of mayonnaise and sour cream.

—Scott Wilson, C.E.C., A.A.C.

Note: We've included bonus recipes in this study's menu plans. Recipes for *italicized* items in menus can be found after each meal-time section.

● BREAKFAST

  1 packet instant Cream of Wheat

  1 slice whole-wheat toast

  1 tsp. reduced-calorie margarine

  1 c. nonfat milk

Exchanges: 2 breads, 1 fruit, 1 milk, ½ fat

~~~~~~

1½ c. Special K cereal

  1 c. nonfat milk

  1 c. sliced strawberries

Exchanges: 2 breads, 1 fruit, 1 milk

~~~~~~

  1 packet Quaker Extra instant oatmeal

  1 slice whole-wheat toast

 ½ medium banana

  1 tsp. peanut butter

  1 c. nonfat milk

Exchanges: 2 breads, 1 fruit, 1 milk, ½ fat

~~~~~~

  1 poached egg (or egg cooked with nonstick cooking spray)

  2 slices whole-wheat toast

  1 small apple

Exchanges: 1 meat, 2 breads, 1 fruit, ½ fat

~~~~~~

  1 small whole-wheat bagel, topped with

  2 tbsp. reduced-calorie cream cheese and

  1 tbsp. all-fruit spread

 ½ grapefruit

 ½ c. nonfat milk

Exchanges: ½ meat, 2 breads, 1 fruit, ½ milk, ½ fat

~~~~~~

1 c. prepared grits, mixed with

1 slice 2% cheddar cheese, diced

½ c. milk

1 small banana

Exchanges: ½ meat, 2 breads, 1 fruit, ½ milk, ½ fat

~~~~~~

½ c. *Low-Fat Granola with Dried Fruit*

½ c. nonfat milk

½ small banana

Exchanges: ½ meat, 2 breads, 1 fruit, ½ milk, 1 fat

~~~~~~

Strawberry-Banana Smoothie

1 slice whole-wheat toast

1 tsp. reduced-calorie margarine

Exchanges: 1 bread, 2 fruits, 1 milk, ½ fat

~~~~~~

Breakfast Burrito

1 c. diced pineapple

Exchanges: 1 meat, 2 breads, 1 fruit, ½ fat

~~~~~~

Grilled Cheese Sandwich

½ c. nonfat milk

½ medium grapefruit

Exchanges: ½ meat, 2 breads, 1 fruit, 1 milk, ½ fat

~~~~~~

2 Sister Schubert (or similar) frozen yeast rolls, baked

2 tsp. all-fruit spread

6 oz. artificially sweetened or plain nonfat yogurt

1 small orange

Exchanges: 2 breads, 1 fruit, 1 milk, ½ fat

~~~~~~

1 medium reduced-fat blueberry muffin

1 medium peach

6 oz. artificially sweetened fruit-flavored nonfat yogurt

Exchanges: 2 breads, 1 fruit, 1 milk, ½ fat

~~~~~~

1 ½ c. multigrain flakes cereal

¾ c. blueberries

1 c. nonfat milk

Exchanges: 2 breads, 1 fruit, 1 milk

~~~~~~

2 low-fat Eggo frozen waffles

½ c. unsweetened applesauce, mixed with

1 packet Splenda sweetener

½ c. sliced strawberries

1 c. nonfat milk

Exchanges: 2 breads, 1 fruit, 1 milk, ½ fat

BONUS BREAKFAST RECIPES

Low-Fat Granola with Dried Fruit

1 c. boiling water

¼ c. dried cranberries

1 6-oz. pkg. dried mixed tropical fruit

2 tbsp. packed brown sugar

3 c. regular oats

¼ c. sliced almonds

¼ c. chopped pecans

¼ c. unsweetened coconut flakes

½ tsp. ground cinnamon

½ tsp. vanilla

Nonstick cooking spray

Preheat oven to 300° F. Combine water, cranberries, tropical fruits and brown sugar in large bowl; mix well and let stand 15 minutes. In large bowl, combine oats, almonds, pecans, coconut flakes, cinnamon and vanilla; blend well and stir into fruit mixture. Spread mixture evenly (about ½ -inch thick) onto two cookie sheets coated with cooking spray. Bake 1 hour, stirring every 15 minutes. Cool to room temperature and store in an airtight container. Makes 12 ½ -cup servings.

Exchanges: ½ meat, 2 breads, ½ fruit, 1 fat

~~~~~~

Strawberry-Banana Smoothie

1   6-oz. artificially sweetened vanilla-flavored low-fat yogurt

½   small banana

2   strawberries, halved and hulled

½   c. orange juice

Combine all ingredients in a blender and blend until smooth. Makes a 1 ½ -cup serving.

Exchanges: 2 fruits, 1 milk

~~~~~~

Breakfast Burrito

2   6-in. fat-free flour tortillas

1   egg

2   tbsp. prepared salsa

Nonstick cooking spray

Heat nonstick skillet; then coat with cooking spray. Scramble egg with salsa; cooking thoroughly. Divide mixture; spoon into tortillas.

Exchanges: 1 meat, 2 breads, ½ fat

~~~~~~

Grilled Cheese Sandwich

2   slices whole-wheat toast

1   slice 2% cheddar cheese

Butter-flavored nonstick cooking spray

Heat nonstick skillet; then coat with cooking spray. Assemble sandwich and grill, turning occasionally to brown both sides. Cook until browned and cheese is melted.

Exchanges: ½ meat, 2 breads, ½ fat

☻ LUNCH

> **Tip**: Enjoy a small green salad (1 cup) with 2 tablespoons fat-free dressing to round out any of these meals—without altering the exchanges.

Burger

1 whole-wheat hamburger bun
1 Classic Boca Burger patty (you can substitute brands if necessary, but make sure the protein for the patty is at least 15 grams)
   Condiments of choice (be sure to check your Member's Guide for added exchanges)
1 c. carrot sticks with
1 tbsp. reduced-fat ranch dressing
1 small apple

Exchanges: 2 meats, 2 breads, 1 vegetable, 1 fruit, 1 fat

~~~~~~

Veggie Pizza

1 7-in. flat-style whole-wheat pita bread
¼ c. *Marinara Sauce* (you can also use prepared marinara sauce)
¼ c. frozen chopped broccoli
¼ c. diced tomatoes
¼ c. sliced mushrooms
¼ c. shredded part-skim Mozzarella cheese

> **Tip**: The vegetables listed are simply suggestions; you can use any combination of vegetables for this great pizza!

Preheat oven to 500° F. Spread marinara on pita bread; top with vegetables and cheese. Bake 5 to 8 minutes or until bread is crisp. Serves 1.

Serve with *Gingered-Fruit Salad*.

Exchanges: 1 meat, 2 breads, 1 vegetable, 1 fruit, 1 fat

~~~~~~

Grilled Veggie Cheese Sandwich

 2 slices multigrain bread
 1 tbsp. reduced-calorie vegetable cream cheese spread
 ½ c. *Grilled Vegetables*
 2 slices reduced-fat Swiss cheese
    Butter-flavored nonstick cooking spray

Preheat nonstick skillet; then coat with cooking spray. Spread cream cheese on one side of bread; top with vegetables, Swiss cheese and remaining slice of bread. Toast on each side until cheese melts.

Serve with 1 cup mixed fresh fruit.

Exchanges: 2 meats, 2 breads, 1 vegetable, 1 fruit, 1 fat

~~~~~~

Meatless Meatball Minestrone

 2 tsp. olive oil
 ¾ c. diced celery
 ½ c. diced bell pepper
 ½ c. diced onion
 ½ c. diced carrots
 3 c. vegetable broth
 1 28-oz. can diced
    tomatoes
 ½ 16-oz. can kidney beans,
    drained (save remaining beans
    for *Quick Vegetarian Chili*)

 1 8-oz. can green beans, drained
 1 tsp. dried (or 1 tbsp. fresh) basil leaves
 1 tbsp. chopped fresh parsley
 ¾ c. dry macaroni
    Meatless Meatballs

Preheat large saucepan; then add oil, celery, bell pepper and onion. Sauté vegetables over medium-high heat until tender. Add carrots and broth; bring to a boil. Add tomatoes, kidney beans, green beans, basil, parsley and macaroni; let simmer 10 to 12 minutes or until pasta is cooked. Add meatballs and let simmer for additional 5 minutes. Serves 4.

Serve each with 15 frozen seedless grapes.

Exchanges: 2½ meats, 2 breads, 1½ vegetables, 1 fruit, ½ fat

~~~~~~

Veggie and Cheese Pasta

1 6-oz. pkg. fettuccine noodles
1 14½-oz. can reduced-sodium vegetable broth
1 16-oz. pkg. frozen mixed broccoli, cauliflower and carrots
1 c. low-fat cottage cheese
¼ c. freshly grated Parmesan cheese
2 tbsp. chopped fresh basil leaves (or 2 tsp. dried leaf basil)
¼ tsp. crushed red pepper flakes
   Salt and black pepper to taste
4 oz. feta cheese, crumbled

Cook pasta according to package directions, omitting fat and using a small amount of salt. Drain and place in large bowl. While pasta is cooking, use medium saucepan to bring broth to a boil; add vegetables and cook until tender. Drain broth from vegetables into small bowl. Return vegetables to saucepan; set aside. Blend cottage cheese with ½ cup of heated broth until smooth; add mixture to vegetables and stir in Parmesan, basil, red pepper, salt and black pepper. Keep mixture warm; add to cooked drained pasta. Stir to coat; top with feta cheese. May be served hot or cold. Serves 4.

Serve each with 1 small banana.
Exchanges: 2 meats, 2 breads, 2 vegetables, 1 fruit, 1 fat

~~~~~~

Meatless Meatball Hoagie

1 6-in. multigrain hoagie bun, sliced
3 *Meatless Meatballs*
¼ c. *Marinara Sauce*
1 oz. provolone cheese, sliced

Heat meatballs in sauce; spoon onto toasted bun; top with provolone and enjoy!

Serve with 1 small orange and 1 cup green salad topped with 2 tablespoons fat-free dressing.
Exchanges: 2 meats, 2 breads, 1 vegetable, 1 fruit, 1 fat

~~~~~~

Spinach and Four-Cheese Pizza

Pizza Dough

2 c. sliced mushrooms

1 medium onion, sliced

1 medium red bell pepper, sliced

3 cloves garlic, minced

1 c. reduced-fat ricotta cheese

½ c. shredded part-skim mozzarella cheese

¼ c. shredded Parmesan cheese

1 10-oz. pkg. frozen low-fat creamed spinach, thawed

2 tbsp. fat-free sour cream

1 tsp. lemon juice

¼ tsp. nutmeg

Salt and pepper to taste

¼ c. crumbled seasoned feta cheese

Butter-flavored nonstick cooking spray

Preheat oven to 400° F. Prebake pizza dough on large pizza pan for 12 to 15 minutes; remove from oven. Preheat nonstick skillet; then coat with cooking spray. Add mushrooms, onions, bell pepper and garlic to skillet; simmer over medium heat 5 minutes or until vegetables are wilted and all liquid is absorbed. In a medium bowl, combine ricotta, mozzarella, Parmesan, creamed spinach, sour cream, lemon juice, nutmeg, salt and pepper; blend well. Spread mixture on pizza crust; top with feta cheese and bake 12 to 15 minutes or until crust is crisp. Cut into 8 pieces. Serves 4.

Serve each with 1 cup watermelon balls.

Exchanges: 2 meats, 2 breads, 1 ½ vegetables, 1 fruit, 1 ½ fats

~ ~

Sloppy Joes

1 12-oz pkg. prebrowned vegetable protein crumbles

4 whole-wheat hamburger buns

2 tsp. olive oil

½ c. chopped onion

½ c. chopped green bell pepper

1 tsp. minced garlic

¾ c. sliced mushrooms, chopped

½ c. catsup

1 tbsp. brown sugar

½ tbsp. brown mustard

½ tsp. celery seeds

½ tsp. chili powder

Salt and pepper to taste

Water if needed to thin

Preheat medium saucepan over medium-high heat; then add oil. Sauté onion, bell pepper, garlic and mushrooms 5 minutes or until tender. Stir in protein crumbles, catsup, brown sugar, brown mustard, celery seeds, chili powder, salt and pepper. Simmer 10 minutes; adjusting seasonings to taste and adding water if needed to thin. Divide evenly and spoon mixture onto heated open-faced buns.

Serve each with 1 small banana.

Exchanges: 2 meats, 2 breads, 1 vegetable, 1 fruit, ½ fat

~~~~~~

Vegetable and Veggie-Sausage Risotto

8 oz. prebrowned sausage-style vegetable protein patties, crumbled

2 cloves garlic, minced

1 small onion, chopped

1 c. sliced mushrooms, chopped

½ tsp. fennel seeds, crushed

¼ tsp. dried thyme leaves

¼ tsp. dried oregano leaves

¼ tsp. ground allspice

1 c. Arborio rice (don't substitute)

4 c. reduced-sodium vegetable broth

2 c. frozen broccoli florets

¼ c. sun-dried tomato bits (*not* packed in oil)

2 tbsp. freshly grated Parmesan cheese

Salt and pepper to taste

Finely chopped parsley for garnish

Olive oil nonstick cooking spray

Tip: This dish can be made ahead of time and refrigerated. Reheat in microwave before serving.

Preheat large saucepan; then coat with cooking spray. Sauté garlic and onion over medium-high heat, 2 to 3 minutes. Add mushrooms and sauté 2 minutes more; stir in fennel seeds, thyme, oregano, allspice and rice; cook, stirring frequently, 2 minutes or until rice begins to brown.

In medium saucepan, heat broth to boiling; reduce heat and keep hot. Add hot broth to rice mixture ½ cup at a time, stirring constantly until broth is absorbed before adding another ½ cup. Continue process, adding ½ cup at a time until rice mixture is creamy (20 to 25 minutes). Add crumbled protein patties, broccoli and tomato bits during last 10 minutes of cooking time; stirring in Parmesan, salt and pepper last. Garnish with parsley. Serves 4.

Serve each with 1 medium peach.

Exchanges: 2 meats, 3 breads, 1 vegetable, 1 fruit, 1 fat

~~~~~~

Taco Bell

1   cheese quesadilla
½   c. salsa mixed with
1   tbsp. fat-free sour cream
1   c. carrot sticks with
¼   c. fat-free ranch dressing
Exchanges: 1 ½ meats, 2 breads, 2 vegetables, 2 fats

~~~~~~

Pizza Hut

2   medium slices Thin 'n' Crispy Veggie Lovers Pizza
    (ask for extra vegetables)
1   side salad (vegetables only), topped with
2   tbsp. fat-free dressing
Exchanges: 2 meats, 3 breads, 1 vegetable, 1 fat

~~~~~~

Quick Vegetarian Chili

2 tsp. olive oil	1 28-oz. can diced tomatoes
2 cloves garlic, minced	1 16-oz. can tomato sauce
1 c. chopped onion	1 tbsp. chili power
1 12-oz. pkg. prebrowned	1 tsp. ground cumin
vegetable protein crumbles	½ tsp. brown sugar
1 ½ 15-oz. cans kidney beans	4 tsp. reduced-fat sour cream

Add oil to preheated medium saucepan. Sauté garlic and onion over medium-high heat until tender; add protein crumbles, kidney beans, tomatoes, tomato sauce, chili powder, cumin and brown sugar. Bring mixture to a boil; reduce heat and simmer 10 minutes. Serves 4.

Serve each with 1 teaspoon sour cream and 1 small apple.
Exchanges: 2 meats, 2 breads, 2 vegetables, 1 fruit, 1 fat

~~~~~~

Layered Black-Bean Tostadas

4 6-in. corn tortillas
1 c. shredded reduced-fat
   Monterey Jack cheese
1 tbsp. diced green chilies
1 15-oz. can seasoned
   refried black beans
2 c. shredded romaine lettuce

2 tbsp. chopped green onions
4 Roma tomatoes, diced
4 tsp. diced avocado
4 tsp. reduced-fat sour cream
   Nonstick cooking spray

> **Tip:** Season regular refried black beans by adding 1 tbsp. freshly chopped cilantro, $\frac{1}{4}$ tsp. ground cumin and 1 tsp. lime juice. Simmer until combined.

Preheat oven to 350° F. Coat tortillas on both sides with cooking spray and arrange on baking sheet. Bake 5 minutes; turn and bake 1 to 2 minutes more or until crisp. Layer each tortilla evenly as follows: cheese, chilies and beans. Garnish with $\frac{1}{2}$ cup lettuce, $\frac{1}{2}$ tablespoon green onions, tomato, 1 teaspoon avocado and 1 teaspoon sour cream. Serves 4.

Serve each with 1 cup *Gingered-Fruit Salad* and 1 cup carrot sticks.
Exchanges: 2 meats, 2 breads, 1 vegetable, 1 fruit, 1 fat

Twice-Baked Potato

1 6-oz. cooked Idaho potato
$\frac{1}{2}$ c. frozen broccoli florets
$\frac{1}{4}$ c. shredded reduced-fat cheddar cheese
3 slices veggie Canadian bacon, chopped
1 tsp. reduced-fat sour cream
1 tsp. reduced-fat butter
   Salt and pepper to taste
$\frac{1}{2}$ c. salsa

Cut potato in half lengthwise; remove and set pulp aside in small bowl. Combine broccoli, cheese, crumbled bacon, sour cream and butter; mix well to blend. Refill potato skins with pulp mixture and top with salsa. Heat more if needed. Serves 1.

Serve with 1 medium pear.
Exchanges: 2 meats, 2 breads, 1 vegetable, 1 fruit, 1 fat

Marinara Sauce

2 medium onions, chopped
6 cloves garlic, minced
1 tbsp. olive oil
2 16-oz. cans diced tomatoes
  with herbs, drained

$\frac{1}{2}$ c. tomato juice
$\frac{1}{4}$ c. tomato paste
2 tsp. lemon juice
$\frac{1}{2}$ tsp. salt
$\frac{1}{4}$ tsp. pepper

Add oil to nonstick skillet; preheat to medium. Sauté garlic and onions over medium heat until tender. Stir in tomatoes, tomato juice and tomato paste; reduce heat and simmer uncovered 20 minutes or until thickened. Stir in lemon juice, salt and pepper. Makes 4 $\frac{1}{2}$-cup servings.
Exchanges: 2 vegetables, $\frac{1}{2}$ fat

~~~~~~

Meatless Meatballs

12 oz. pkg. prebrowned vegetable
  protein crumbles
1 egg, slightly beaten
$\frac{1}{3}$ c. dry Italian-style bread crumbs
$\frac{1}{4}$ c. all-purpose flour
$\frac{1}{4}$ c. shredded reduced-fat
  Italian-blend cheese

$\frac{1}{4}$ c. minced onion
$\frac{1}{4}$ c. minced green bell pepper
1 clove garlic, minced
$\frac{1}{2}$ tsp. dried oregano leaves
$\frac{1}{2}$ tsp. black pepper
  Nonstick cooking spray

Combine all ingredients in a large bowl; mix well. Preheat oven to 350° F. Form mixture into about 20 meatballs and place onto cookie sheet coated with cooking spray and bake for 12 to 15 minutes or until browned. Makes 4 servings of 5 meatballs.
Exchanges: 2 meats, 1 bread

~~~~~~

Gingered-Fruit Salad

2 tbsp. orange juice
$\frac{1}{4}$ tsp. ground (or 1 tsp.
  freshly grated) ginger
1 c. sliced strawberries

$\frac{1}{2}$ c. each honeydew and
  cantaloupe balls
$\frac{1}{2}$ c. each seedless white
  and red grapes

Combine juice and ginger in medium bowl; add strawberries, melon balls and grapes. Toss to coat; refrigerate until ready to serve. Serves 4.

Exchanges: 1 fruit

~~~~~~

Grilled Vegetables

1 small eggplant, peeled and sliced into ½-in. sections

1 medium zucchini, cut into ½-in. diagonal slices

6 medium mushroom caps, halved

1 medium summer squash, sliced into ½-in. "moons"

2 medium tomatoes, each cut into 6 wedges

1 medium red onion, cut into 6 wedges

½ c. low-calorie Italian dressing

1 tbsp. soy sauce

Salt and pepper to taste

Salt eggplant and set aside (to draw out bitterness). Prepare remaining vegetables. Rinse eggplant and combine with other vegetables in large bowl. Drizzle with Italian dressing, soy sauce, salt and pepper. Let marinate for 20 to 30 minutes while preheating grill to medium-high heat (or while preheating oven to 400° F). Place drained marinated vegetables in grill basket and grill to desired doneness (if using oven, arrange vegetables on baking sheet and bake to desired doneness). Serve hot or cold. Makes 6 1-cup servings.

Exchanges: 2 vegetables, ½ fat

~~~~~~

Pizza Dough

¾ c. all-purpose flour, divided

1 pkg. rapid-rise yeast

¼ tsp. salt

½ c. very hot water

2 tsp. honey

½ c. whole-wheat flour

Combine all-purpose flour, yeast and salt in medium bowl; add hot water and honey, stirring until smooth. Mix in enough whole-wheat flour to make a soft dough. Knead dough on floured surface until smooth and elastic (about 3 to 4 minutes). Cover dough with bowl and let rise 15 minutes. Spread dough and use according to directions for pizza recipes. Makes one 12-inch crust. Cut into 8 slices. Serving size: 2 slices.

Exchanges: 2 breads

✿ DINNER

Lentil and Bulgur Stew

1 c. dried green lentils	2 c. diced eggplant
1 bay leaf	2 vegan soy burgers,
4½ c. water	cut into strips
½ c. bulgur	1 8-oz. can of tomato sauce
½ tsp. salt	1 c. chopped greens (kale,
½ tsp. pepper	collards, mustard greens)
2 tbsp. olive oil	Water, if needed
1 large onion, chopped	
4 to 6 garlic cloves, chopped	

In a large pot, bring lentils, bay leaf and water to a simmer over medium heat. Cook for about 25 minutes; then add bulgur, salt and pepper. Cook, stirring frequently, 15 to 20 minutes more or until lentils are tender, adding a little water if needed.

While lentils are cooking, sauté onion, garlic and eggplant until onions are soft and a little brown, adding a little water if mixture becomes too dry. Add tomato sauce and greens; heat until greens are wilted and tender. Remove from heat; add lentil and bulgur mix. Serve immediately. Serves 4.

Serve each with 1 cup green salad and 2 tablespoons fat-free dressing.
Exchanges: 2½ meats, 2½ breads, 1½ vegetables, 1 fat

~~~~~~

Tofu Goulash

1 lb. frozen firm low-fat tofu,	4 small potatoes, unpeeled,
thawed, crumbled or cut	scrubbed and cut into chunks
into chunks	1 tbsp. sweet paprika
4 tsp. olive oil, divided	1 to 2 c. vegetable broth
1 medium yellow onion, sliced	½ c. frozen green peas
1 8-oz. pkg. sliced mushrooms	Salt and pepper to taste

Brown tofu in 2 teaspoons oil preheated in skillet, adding salt and pepper to taste. Once browned, remove from skillet and set aside. Add remaining 2 teaspoons oil to skillet, heat and sauté onion 5 to 8 minutes or until golden in color; then add mushrooms. When mushrooms begin to throw off their water, add potatoes, stirring constantly. When water from mushrooms is almost fully evaporated stir in paprika, blending well. Add broth; simmer on low heat until potatoes are soft; then add peas and browned tofu. Test for seasoning and allow to simmer until peas are cooked through. Serves 4.

Serve each with ½ cup steamed green beans.

Exchanges: 2½ meats, 1½ breads, 2 vegetables, 1 fat

~~~~~~

Teriyaki Mock Chicken

1 3-oz. Success Brown Rice	2 tsp. olive oil
Boil-in-Bag (10-minute style)	1 c. frozen broccoli florets
1 6-oz. pkg. mock-chicken strips	1 c. frozen cauliflowerets
½ c. teriyaki 10-minute marinade,	1 c. carrot rounds
divided	

Cook rice according to package directions. In small bowl, combine mock-chicken strips and ¼ cup marinade; set aside. Use oil to sauté vegetables in skillet until tender-crisp; add remaining marinade. Sauté 1 minute more; then add mock-chicken strips. Cook until heated through and serve immediately over rice. Serves 2.

Serve each with 1 cup green salad and 2 tablespoons fat-free dressing.

Exchanges: 2 meats, 1½ breads, 2 vegetables, 1½ fats

~~~~~~

Vegetable Omelet

¼ c. julienne carrots	½ c. fat-free egg substitute
¼ c. julienne zucchini	2 tsp. water
¼ c. part-skim ricotta cheese	Pinch salt and black pepper
1 tsp. chopped chives	Nonstick cooking spray

Combine carrots and zucchini in microwave-safe bowl; cover and microwave 2 minutes. Add ricotta and chives to vegetables; set aside. Preheat small nonstick skillet; then coat with cooking spray. Combine egg substitute, water, salt and pepper in small bowl; add to heated skillet. As mixture starts to cook, gently lift edges of omelet with spatula, tilting back and forth until cooked through. Spoon vegetable mixture over half of omelet and fold omelet in half. Serves 1.

Serve with *Sweet Potato Fries.*

Exchanges: 2 meats, 2 breads, 2 vegetables, 1½ fats

~~~~~~

Mock-Crab Cakes

7 slices whole-wheat bread, torn into large pieces	1/4 c. chopped parsley
1 tbsp. canola oil	16 oz. firm, regular tofu, pressed
3/4 c. minced celery	1 tsp. salt
3/4 c. chopped white onion	2 tbsp. Old Bay seasoning
1/2 c. minced carrot	1/2 c. low-fat mayonnaise
1 small green pepper, minced	1 egg
	Nonstick cooking spray

Preheat oven to 350° F. In a food processor or blender, whirl bread pieces into fine crumbs. Place on a baking sheet and bake 8 to 10 minutes or until dried and toasty. Remove from oven and set aside. Heat medium skillet; then add oil and sauté celery, onion, carrot, pepper and parsley 5 minutes or until softened. Remove from heat and set aside. Use food processor or blender to pulse tofu to cottage-cheese consistency—being very careful not to puree. Combine tofu, sautéed vegetables, 1/2 cup bread crumbs, salt, Old Bay seasoning, mayonnaise and egg. Mix well and refrigerate for 1 hour.

Form chilled mixture into 8 patties, each about 3 inches across and 1/2-inch thick (about 1/2 cup for each). Coat each patty with remaining bread crumbs; place on nonstick baking sheet coated with cooking spray. Spray patty tops lightly with cooking spray; bake 15 minutes at 350° F; carefully turn over and bake 10 minutes more or until toasted and brown. Serves 4.

Serve each with 2 tablespoons *Fat-Free Remoulade Sauce* and 1 serving of *Broccoli au Gratin*.

Exchanges: 3 meats, 2 breads, 2 vegetables, 1 1/2 fats

~~~~~~

Beef-Style Stroganoff

4 oz. uncooked egg noodles	2 tbsp. all-purpose flour
1 tbsp. olive oil	1 15 3/4 -oz. can French onion soup
1 medium onion, chopped	1 tsp. Worcestershire sauce
1 garlic clove, minced	1 c. reduced-fat sour cream
4 oz. mushrooms, sliced	Pepper to taste
4 vegan soy burgers, cut into strips	

Prepare noodles according to package directions omitting fat. Use olive oil to sauté garlic and onion in medium skillet 2 to 3 minutes. Add mushrooms and soy strips; continue to sauté until browned. Sprinkle flour over mixture and sauté 1 minute more; slowly add soup until mixture thickens. Add Worcestershire sauce and let cool slightly. Stir in sour cream and adjust seasonings as desired. Spoon over egg noodles to serve. Serves 4.

Serve each with 1 serving *Cauliflower au Gratin*.
Exchanges: 2½ meats, 2 breads, 2 vegetables, 1½ fats

~~~~~~

Stouffer's 9 ⅛-oz. Lean Cuisine Cheese Cannelloni

Prepare as directed. Serves 1.

Serve with 1 slice garlic breadstick and 1 serving *Sautéed Greens*.
Exchanges: 1½ meats, 2½ breads, 2 vegetables, 1 fat

~~~~~~

Shepherd's Pie

1 12-oz. pkg. prebrowned soy-burger crumbles	Salt and pepper (to taste)
1 large white onion, diced	3 large russet potatoes
2 tbsp. all-purpose flour	½ c. nonfat milk
⅔ c. water	2 tbsp. reduced-fat butter
1 tsp. Kitchen Bouquet gravy seasoning	

In a large skillet, brown soy crumbles (oil can be used sparingly to prevent sticking). Remove from heat; add onion, flour, water and gravy seasoning; salt and pepper to taste. Mix well; place mixture in casserole dish and set aside. Peel and cook potatoes; drain and add margarine, milk; salt and pepper to taste. Mash potatoes; then place on top of soy-crumble mixture in casserole dish.

Broil uncovered 10 to 15 minutes or until topping is browned. (Note: If dish is not heated thoroughly before topping is browned, you can bake or microwave further to heat through.) Serves 4.

Serve each with 1 cup *Grilled Vegetables* (see the bonus recipes for lunches).
Exchanges: 2 meats, 2 breads, 2 vegetables, 1 fat

~~~~~~

Mediterranean-Style Macaroni and Cheese

1 10-oz. Stouffer's Lean Cuisine Macaroni and Cheese, thawed	$\frac{1}{4}$ c. diced carrots
$\frac{1}{2}$ tsp. olive oil	$\frac{1}{2}$ c. chopped baby spinach leaves
$\frac{1}{4}$ tbsp. chopped onion	1 Roma tomato, diced
$\frac{1}{4}$ tbsp. chopped bell pepper	$\frac{1}{2}$ tsp. dried leaf oregano
	2 oz. reduced-fat feta cheese with herbs

Preheat medium skillet; add oil, onion, bell pepper and carrots; sauté until tender. Add spinach and tomato; sauté 2 minutes more or until spinach is completely wilted. Combine in large microwave-safe bowl with thawed macaroni and cheese, oregano and feta cheese. Divide mixture in half (to heat evenly) and microwave 2 to 3 minutes or until hot. Serves 2.

Serve each with 1 cup steamed green beans.

Exchanges: 2 meats, 2 breads, 2 vegetables, $\frac{1}{2}$ skim milk, 1 fat

~~~~~~

Greek-Style Casserole

6 oz. uncooked penne pasta	1 pkg. veggie Canadian bacon, julienne
$\frac{1}{2}$ c. crumbled feta cheese, divided	1 14$\frac{1}{2}$-oz. can diced tomatoes
2 tsp. olive oil	$\frac{1}{4}$ c. chopped ripe olives
4 c. peeled, cubed eggplant	$\frac{1}{4}$ tsp. Italian seasoning
2 tsp. salt	Nonstick cooking spray
1 c. chopped purple onion	

Cook pasta according to package directions, omitting salt and fat; drain. Place cooked pasta in 11x7x2-inch baking dish coated with cooking spray. Sprinkle with $\frac{1}{4}$ cup feta cheese and set aside. Preheat oven to 350° F. Sprinkle eggplant with salt and let sit for 10 to 15 minutes to remove bitterness; then rinse thoroughly and pat dry. Preheat nonstick skillet and sauté eggplant and onion in oil over medium-high heat 5 minutes or until tender. Stir in remaining ingredients except cheese. Cover, reduce heat and simmer 3 to 4 minutes; then pour over pasta and sprinkle with remaining cheese. Bake 15 minutes; serve hot. Serves 4.

Serve each with 1 cup green salad and 2 tablespoons fat-free dressing.

Exchanges: 2 meats, 2 breads, 2 vegetables, 1$\frac{1}{2}$ fats

~~~~~~

Broccoli "Beef" Stir-Fry

2 soy-protein patties
2 tsp. vegetable oil, divided
2 c. broccoli florets
¼ tsp. ground ginger
1 garlic clove, minced

1 c. condensed tomato soup
1 tbsp. cider vinegar
1 tsp. soy sauce
1½ c. hot cooked brown rice

Slice soy patties into ½-inch strips. Preheat medium-sized nonstick skillet; then add 1 teaspoon oil and stir-fry soy strips over high heat 1 minute or until browned. Once browned, remove from skillet and set aside. Reduce heat; add remaining oil and stir-fry broccoli florets until tender-crisp. Stir in ginger, garlic, soup, vinegar and soy sauce; heat to boiling. Stir in soy strips; heat through and serve over rice. Serves 2.

Serve each with 1 serving *Collard Greens with Tomatoes.*
Exchanges: 2½ meats, 3 breads, 2 vegetables, 1 fat

~~~~~~

Chinese Veggie Stir-Fry

¼ c. fresh lemon juice
2 tbsp. soy sauce
2 tbsp. water
1 tbsp. freshly grated gingerroot
   (or ½ tsp. ground ginger)
1 tsp. sugar
2 garlic cloves, minced
1 16-oz. firm low-fat tofu,
   drained, pressed and cubed
3 c. cooked brown rice

1 c. chopped onion
1½ tbsp. olive oil
2 c. shredded Chinese cabbage
1 c. fresh bean sprouts
1 c. diced sweet red pepper
1 c. sliced fresh mushrooms
1 c. snow peas
¼ c. green onions, sliced diagonally
2 tsp. cornstarch

Combine lemon juice, soy sauce, water, ginger, sugar and garlic in large bowl. Add tofu and onion; cover and marinate in refrigerator 2 to 3 hours. Drain and reserve marinade. Preheat large nonstick skillet over medium-high heat; then add oil and tofu mixture. Stir-fry 5 minutes or until tofu begins to brown; then remove mixture and set aside. Add cabbage, bean sprouts, red pepper, mushrooms, snow peas and green onions to skillet; stir-fry 2 to 3 minutes or until vegetables are tender-crisp. Combine reserved marinade with cornstarch, stirring well. Add marinade and simmer 2 minutes or until thickened; then add tofu and simmer 1 to 2 minutes more. Arrange equal servings over ¾ cup rice. Serves 4.

Exchanges: 2½ meats, 2 breads, 2 vegetables, 1 fat

~~~~~~

Italian Skillet Dinner

2 tsp. olive oil
1 c. chopped zucchini
½ c. sliced onion
½ c. sliced celery
½ c. diced red bell pepper
1 tsp. dried oregano
2 garlic cloves, minced
1 14½-oz. can diced
 tomatoes, drained

1 12-oz. pkg. Italian-flavored
 vegetable crumbles
1 15-oz. can cannellini (or other
 white beans), rinsed and drained
2 rosemary sprigs
1 c. freshly chopped baby spinach
½ c. shredded part-skim mozzarella
 cheese
⅛ tsp. black pepper

Preheat large nonstick skillet over medium-high heat; then add oil and sauté zucchini, onion, celery, bell pepper oregano and garlic 2 minutes. Stir in tomatoes, vegetable crumbles, beans and rosemary; cook 2 minutes more. Add spinach, cheese and black pepper; cook 1 minute more or until spinach wilts and cheese begins to melt. Discard rosemary. Serves 4.

Serve each with 1 serving *Marinated Asparagus.*

Exchanges: 3 meats, 2 breads, 2 vegetables, 1½ fats

~~~~~~

Spaghetti Frittata

1 c. cooked spaghetti
 (about 2 oz. uncooked)
2 tbsp. freshly chopped parsley
1 tbsp. freshly chopped basil
1 tsp. freshly chopped tarragon
½ tsp. freshly chopped rosemary
2 oz. fat-free cream cheese, chilled
 and cut into small pieces

¼ tsp. black pepper
1 c. egg substitute
3 garlic cloves, minced
6 ¼-in. slices Roma tomato
¼ c. grated Asiago cheese
 Nonstick cooking spray

Preheat oven to 450° F. Combine spaghetti, parsley, basil, tarragon, rosemary, cream cheese, pepper and egg substitute in large bowl; stir well and set aside. Coat a 10-inch nonstick skillet with cooking spray; place over medium heat until hot. Add garlic; sauté 3 minutes. Stir in spaghetti mixture; spread evenly in bottom of skillet. Cook over medium-low heat 5 minutes or until almost set. Arrange tomato slices over top; sprinkle with Asiago cheese. Wrap handle of skillet with foil; place skillet in oven and bake 5 minutes or until set. Serves 2.

Serve each with 1 serving *Tabbouleh.*

Exchanges: 2½ meats, 2 breads, 2½ vegetables, 1½ fats

~~~~~~

BONUS DINNER RECIPES

Sweet Potato Fries

1 medium sweet potato,
  peeled and cut into
  4x½-inch thick fries

½ tsp. olive oil
2 tsp. balsamic vinegar
Salt and pepper to taste

Preheat oven to 375° F. Coat fries with olive oil; place on baking sheet and bake 20 to 25 minutes. Drizzle with vinegar; bake additional 5 to 10 minutes. Sprinkle with salt and pepper. Serves 1.

Exchanges: 2 breads, ½ fat

~~~~~~

Fat-Free Remoulade Sauce

1 c. fat-free mayonnaise
2 tbsp. country-style mustard
1 tbsp. dill-pickle relish
1 tsp. horseradish

1 tsp. capers
1 tsp. lemon juice
½ tsp. paprika

Combine all ingredients in small bowl; refrigerate until needed. Makes 8 servings of 2 tablespoons each.

Exchanges: None! It's a free food.

~~~~~~

Broccoli au Gratin

¼ c. seasoned bread crumbs
1 10-oz. pkg. frozen chopped broccoli, thawed
¼ c. egg substitute
2 oz. shredded reduced-fat cheddar cheese
  Salt and pepper to taste
  Nonstick cooking spray

Preheat oven to 350° F. Combine all ingredients in small bowl; mix well. Spoon into small baking dish coated with cooking spray and bake 15 minutes. Serves 2.

Exchanges: 1 meat, ½ bread, 1 vegetable, ½ fat

~~~~~~

Cauliflower au Gratin

3 c. frozen cauliflowerets

1 tsp. butter

1 tsp. flour

1 c. nonfat milk

¼ c. shredded reduced-fat cheddar cheese

Place cauliflowerets in a microwave-safe dish and microwave, covered, 3 to 4 minutes or until thawed. Drain off any excess water and set aside. Melt butter in small saucepan over low heat. Whisk flour and milk together in microwave-safe bowl; microwave 1 minute. Slowly add milk mixture to butter, whisking continuously over low heat until thickened. Add cheese and whisk until completely melted. Add cheese sauce to cauliflower; heat 2 minutes in microwave and serve hot. Serves 4.

Exchanges: ½ meat, 1 vegetable, ½ fat

~~~~~~

Cheesy Collard Greens with Tomatoes

1 large bunch collard greens, stems and ribs removed

1 tbsp. olive oil

2 garlic cloves, chopped

1 28-oz. can diced tomatoes

1 tsp. salt

1 tsp. oregano

4 oz. reduced-fat cheddar cheese, shredded

Bring large pot of water to rolling boil; add greens and cook 10 minutes or until tender. Drain and roughly chop; set aside. Heat oil in large skillet; add garlic and sauté 1 minute. Add greens, tomatoes, salt and oregano; cook 4 to 5 minutes more. Top with shredded cheese prior to serving. Serves 4.

Exchanges: 1 meat, 1 vegetable, ½ fat

~~~~~~

Sautéed Greens

2 tsp. olive oil
1 medium onion, diced
1 large bunch fresh greens (kale, collards, turnips or mustard greens),
   washed, cleaned and chopped (or 1 lb. frozen, thawed)
¼ c. vegetable broth
1 tbsp. balsamic vinegar

Sauté onion in large skillet over medium heat until tender. Add
chopped greens, broth and vinegar; continue to sauté 8 to 10 minutes or until tender. Serves 4.
Exchanges: 1 vegetable

~~~~~~

Marinated Asparagus

2 lbs. asparagus spears, tough ends removed
½ c. reduced-fat raspberry vinaigrette salad dressing

Steam asparagus 3 to 4 minutes or until tender. Place in small dish and
drizzle with dressing; refrigerate until chilled. Serves 4.
Exchanges: 1 vegetable, ½ fat

~~~~~~

Tabbouleh

¼ c. uncooked bulgur
   (cracked wheat)
1 tbsp. fresh lemon juice
2 tsp. olive oil
¼ c. finely chopped
   green onions
1 garlic clove, minced

1 c. finely chopped Roma tomato
¾ c. finely chopped celery
⅓ c. finely chopped fresh parsley
½ c. finely chopped seeded cucumber
¼ tsp. salt

Combine bulgur, lemon juice and olive oil in 2-quart bowl; stir well.
Layer green onions, garlic, tomato, celery, parsley and cucumber in
order over bulgur mixture; sprinkle salt over cucumber. Cover and
chill 24 hours. Serves 2.
Exchanges: ½ bread, 1 ½ vegetables, ½ fat

CONVERSION CHART
EQUIVALENT IMPERIAL AND METRIC MEASUREMENTS

Liquid Measures

Fluid Ounces	U.S.	Imperial	Milliliters
	1 teaspoon	1 teaspoon	5
$\frac{1}{4}$	2 teaspoons	1 dessert spoon	7
$\frac{1}{2}$	1 tablespoon	1 tablespoon	15
1	2 tablespoons	2 tablespoons	28
2	$\frac{1}{4}$ cup	4 tablespoons	56
4	$\frac{1}{2}$ cup or $\frac{1}{4}$ pint		110
5		$\frac{1}{4}$ pint or 1 gill	140
6	$\frac{3}{4}$ cup		170
8	1 cup or $\frac{1}{2}$ pint		225
9			250 or $\frac{1}{4}$ liter
10	$1\frac{1}{4}$ cups	$\frac{1}{2}$ pint	280
12	$1\frac{1}{2}$ cups or $\frac{3}{4}$ pint		340
15		3/4 pint	420
16	2 cups or 1 pint		450
18	$2\frac{1}{4}$ cups		500 or $\frac{1}{2}$ liter
20	$2\frac{1}{2}$ cups	1 pint	560
24	3 cups or $1\frac{1}{2}$ pints		675
25		$1\frac{1}{4}$	700
30	$3\frac{3}{4}$ cups	$1\frac{1}{2}$ pints	840
32	4 cups		900
36	$4\frac{1}{2}$ cups		1000 or 1 liter
40	5 cups	2 pints or 1 quart	1120
48	6 cups or 3 pints		1350
50		$2\frac{1}{2}$ pints	1400

Solid Measures

U.S. and Imperial Measures		Metric Measures	
Ounces	Pounds	Grams	Kilos
1		28	
2		56	
3½		100	
4	¼	112	
5		140	
6		168	
8	½	225	
9		250	¼
12	¾	340	
16	1	450	
18		500	½
20	1¼	560	
24		675	
27		750	¾
32	2	900	
36	2¼	1000	1
40	2½	1100	
48	3	1350	
54		1500	1½
64	4	1800	
72	4½	2000	2
80	5	2250	2¼
100	6	2800	2¾

Oven Temperature Equivalents

Fahrenheit	Celsius	Gas Mark	Description
225	110	1/4	Cool
250	130	1/2	
275	140	1	Very Slow
300	150	2	
325	170	3	Slow
350	180	4	Moderate
375	190	5	
400	200	6	Moderately Hot
425	220	7	Fairly Hot
450	230	8	Hot
475	240	9	Very Hot
500	250	10	Extremely Hot

LEADER'S DISCUSSION GUIDE

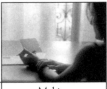

Week One: God's Command

1. **Before the meeting**: Set two place settings on a table in the front of the room. On one plate, place a card on which you've written "Life"; on the other plate, set a card on which you've written "Death." Make sure these labels can be read by everyone in the room.

2. Begin the meeting by having everyone say the memory verse in unison. Discuss: Why do you think God did not just tell us what to do, rather than give us a choice? Ask members to share positives and negatives of being allowed to choose freely. Point to the table settings and remind members that they each must make the choice between life and death.

3. Invite a volunteer to read Deuteronomy 28:2. Discuss why God puts a prerequisite on His blessings for us.

4. Bring a walnut or other nut and a hammer or heavy object. Have members compare their enemy in their current struggle with weight loss or bad habits. Smash the nut and explain: This is how God will destroy the hold the enemy has on you. Feel the freedom in your life as the enemy is scattered.

5. Read Deuteronomy 28:9. Have someone look up or provide a definition of "oath." Form two groups, and have one group discuss God's part in an oath and the other group discuss our part in the oath. Allow 8 to 10 minutes for discussion. Bring the whole group back together. Discuss the benefits of obedience to God.

6. Have each member write a goal on paper along with several obstacles to reaching that goal. Read Deuteronomy 28:8, then form a standing circle. One by one—being considerate of members who may not feel like praying aloud—have members pray a prayer of obedience, with you closing the prayer. Ask God to take the needs expressed and bring each member victory as they follow Him in obedience.

Week Two: The Balanced Life

1. Display an enlarged picture of the First Place logo. Have members explain the meaning of the four parts of the balanced life.

2. Read Luke 2:41-47. Form four groups, and assign each group one of the following words or phrases: "Listening," "Ask Questions," "Gain Understanding," "Provide Answers." Discuss how each of these four steps can help us grow mentally and benefit us in the First Place program.

3. Have someone read Proverbs 31:17. Then ask a volunteer to recite Luke 2:52 from memory. Invite another volunteer to write words on the board or a large sheet of paper. Brainstorm activities done in child-hood. Allow five minutes of fast and furious brainstorming. When the five minutes is up, circle any listed activities that members feel they can incorporate into their daily and weekly First Place program.

4. Have a member read James 1:4. Discuss what spiritual maturity is. Role-play a conversation between Janet and Leigh. Janet is spiritually mature, and Leigh has not been in a Bible study for many years. They are discussing the benefits of a daily quiet time. Janet helps Leigh come to understand how she can make better choices by spending time alone with God every day.

5. Ask two volunteers to do the following role-play: Debi is having friends over for brunch and a swim at her home. Jackie did not receive an invitation and is hurt. Have Jackie respond first in a negative way when she sees Debi in church the next day. Have her use body language as well as verbal responses. Then repeat the scene and have her respond in a positive way.

6. Read Revelation 1:17. Point out the cross at the end of the word "First" in the logo. Explain: If we put Christ first in all four areas, we will have proper balance in our lives. We can choose to allow Jesus to supply all our needs and change our unhealthy habits, or we can continue old ones and our sedentary lifestyle. Remind members: It is all about *making wise choices.*

7. Close with a prayer for proper balance in our lives, putting Jesus Christ in the center.

Week Three: Doing It All

1. Recite this week's memory verse in unison.

2. Before the meeting: Select a recipe and remove some items from the list of ingredients. Make copies for everyone. Explain: Let's review the ingredients. Read through it. Ask: Do you think this recipe will be a success? Discuss what happens when we only obey partially.

3. Read Joshua 11:11. Discuss how members felt as they completed the activity on Day 2, page 35, in which the listed foods they should eliminate from their kitchen.

4. Discuss some of the other things they should eliminate from their lives (e.g., ugly habits such as gossip, grudge holding, bad attitudes, etc.).

5. Ask members to name some kings that reign in their lives. Suggest one or two if necessary.

6. Select one of the "kings" and walk through the dethroning steps (p. 37) on the board or a large sheet of paper.

7. Read Joshua 24:19-22 aloud. Discuss how understanding God's jealous feelings for us might help us in First Place.

10. Read Joshua 11:23 and pray that God will relieve weary hearts and give rest from war.

Week Four: Action Brings Hope

1. Invite a volunteer (or two) to share a time when they became frustrated at trying to resolve a problem and were unable to reach the person with the authority to solve it. Discuss how they felt and reacted.

2. Explain that before something becomes an action, it must begin as a thought in the mind. Discuss: How can we can prepare our minds as we continue our journey to a better life?

3. Form three groups and assign each group one of the following verses: Matthew 11:28; 1 Corinthians 9:25; 1 Corinthians 10:31. Direct each group to select a spokesperson to share the key thought from their Scripture passage and how it applies to First Place.

4. Ask a volunteer to share what their quiet time is like.

5. Read Matthew 5:44. Explain the meaning of "sandpaper people." Discuss: How can we love people who rub us the wrong way?

6. Have members think about some of the sandpaper people in their own lives. Form a circle of prayer, asking God to love others through each member in the circle.

7. Ask a volunteer to recite 1 Peter 1:13 from memory.

8. Discuss: What is the grace given to us?

9. Do not allow this class to close without encouraging members who may not know Jesus Christ to do so.

Week Five: A Discerning Heart

1. Have a volunteer recite this week's memory verse. Or do it in unison.

2. Ask for examples of wanting good things for the wrong reasons. Discuss why it might or might not be wrong.

3. Invite volunteers to share some insight God has given them about discernment from Day 1.

4. Read Proverbs 1:2-6 and discuss the purpose of wisdom.

5. On the board or a large sheet of paper, write the phrase, "Knowing What to Choose" on the left side and on the other side write "Unfaithfulness." Have members call out examples for each column (e.g., having daily quiet time versus rushing out the door; exercising versus ignoring it; cooking healthy meals versus running out for fast food). Discuss the wisdom in doing what is right.

6. Discuss: What is the secret of extending the length of your life? Discuss 1 Kings 3:14 and how to apply it to our life today.

7. Have members share how memorizing Scripture has helped them in their First Place journey. If anyone expresses difficulty in memorizing, invite suggestions from the group. Encourage them to try the First Place Scripture CDs in the back of the study.

8. Close with a prayer of commitment to obedience and a prayer of thankfulness for God's measureless blessings.

Week Six: Everything Permissible

1. Have several volunteers recite this week's memory verse.

2. Read John 8:32 and discuss how to "hold to His teachings."

3. Form two groups. On the board or a large sheet of paper, write "Name It" on the left side and "Deal with It" on the right. Have members of one group call out things that might control a person (e.g., food, spending, anger, etc.).

4. Have members of the second group provide a list of alternatives to the things listed on the board.

5. Ask a member to look up "temple" in a dictionary and read the definition. Ask members to suggest ways to treat their body as a temple.

6. **Before the meeting**: Find a pretty vase or a picture of something valuable and bring it to the meeting. Display it at this time. Share with members the importance of taking care of that which is valuable. Make the comparison between that and our body as a temple.

7. Invite members to share ways they have chosen to honor God with their bodies. Identify which side—physical, mental, spiritual or emotional—it represents.

8. Close in prayer asking God to encourage members to treat their bodies as something valuable and to help members choose healthy things in caring for their bodies.

Week Seven: Rebuilding Your Life

1. **Before the meeting**: Write each of the four steps (p. 79) on a separate index card.

2. Have a volunteer read Haggai 1:8. Form four groups and give one card to each group. Give them five minutes to discuss ways to put their step into action in making lifestyle changes.

3. Call small groups back. Begin with a call for their reports, listing two or three suggestions for each step on the board or a large sheet of paper.

4. Read Haggai 2:9. Ask members to think of their new body as God's temple. Invite them to share what would be different in their lives if they lived like they are God's temple.

5. Close with a prayer that God will help each individual to rebuild their body.

Week Eight: Two Kinds of Wisdom

1. Recite James 3:13 in unison. Form two teams: Heavenly Wisdom and Earthly Wisdom.

2. Have a member of the Earthly Wisdom team read James 3:14-16 aloud. Give them five minutes to give examples of earthly wisdom: envy, selfish ambition, boastfulness, denial of truth, disorder and evil practices.

3. Discuss possible consequences of earthly wisdom and list alternatives for each.

4. Read James 3:17.

5. Ask the Heavenly Wisdom team to give examples of using heavenly wisdom in the First Place program, giving them five minutes.

6. Discuss the biblical models of heavenly wisdom.

7. Have one member of the Heavenly Wisdom team read Philippians 2:3.

8. Discuss why humility is important in the First Place program.

9. Remind the class that heavenly wisdom comes from Christ and earthly wisdom draws on the worldly system.

10. Ask a member from each team to pray for heavenly wisdom to make wise choices.

Week Nine: The Right or the Wrong Help

1. Read Psalm 20:7.

2. Discuss: What are some reasons we seek help from places and things other than God? Have a volunteer record the reasons on the board or a large sheet of paper.

3. Remind them that the Israelites did not want to pay the price of seeking God's help. Discuss: What price do we pay for seeking God's help? What must we do? Why might we not be willing to pay the price?

4. Share an inner struggle you may have had and how it contributed to your weight problem. Invite others to share their struggle. Discuss ways to deal with it.

5. Have members share obstacles to success in First Place while you write them on the board or a large sheet of paper. After all have been listed, draw a big red X through them and write "GOD" over the list. Assure members that God's power is mightier than a horseman's strength.

6. Read Isaiah 30:18-21 aloud.

7. Discuss the ways that God is gracious and compassionate toward us.

8. Invite volunteers to share their answers to the personal questions on Day 5. Be sensitive to those who may not feel comfortable about sharing aloud.

9. Close with a prayer circle and ask for God's guidance in choosing the right help—His help.

Week Ten: The Most Important Choice

1. In unison, recite John 3:16.

2. Give members a sheet of paper and a pen or pencil each and ask them to list the people for whom they would give their life.

3. Discuss the fact that even if they did die for a spouse or child, they could not provide eternal life.

4. Read Hebrews 10:17-18.

5. Explain how Jesus died on the cross to pay for all our sins, past, present and future. Emphasize that He only had to die once and that He would have done it to save just one person.

6. Discuss: How many of you have forgiven someone for a wrong but cannot seem to forget it? Make the point that Jesus forgets our sin once it has been confessed and forgiven. Share Psalm 103:12.

7. Refer back to the week one study about choosing between life and death. Ask a volunteer to say the week one memory verse. Read John 3:36 and compare it with Deuteronomy 30:19. Remind members that God provides us with a choice and that this study is about making wise choices.

8. Read 2 Peter 3:9 from page 119. Discuss: Why do you think God is patient with those who have not believed in Him?

9. Discuss the word "perish" and what it means. Discuss: How might disobedience to God result in death?

10. Discuss: What can we do when we know we have been disobedient? (Confess, ask for and receive forgiveness from God; see 1 John 1:9).

11. Discuss the key thoughts of the Scriptures on Day 5. Share the ABCs of salvation from page 121. Explain: If you already know Jesus as your personal Lord and Savior, this might be a good time to recommit your life to Him. If you have never trusted Him for eternal life, now would be a wonderful time to do so.

12. Close with the prayer of salvation for the lost and a recommitment of lives to serve God in a healthy body.

PERSONAL WEIGHT RECORD

Week	Weight	+ or -	Goal This Session	Pounds to Goal
1				
2				
3				
4				
5				
6				
7				
8				
9				
10				
11				
12				
13				
Final				

Beginning Measurements

Waist_____ Hips_____ Thighs_____ Chest_____

Ending Measurements

Waist_____ Hips_____ Thighs_____ Chest_____

COMMITMENT RECORDS

How to Fill Out a Commitment Record

The Commitment Record (CR) is an aid for you in keeping track of your accomplishments. Begin a new CR on the morning of the day your class meets. This ensures that your CR is complete before your next meeting. Turn in the CR weekly to your leader.

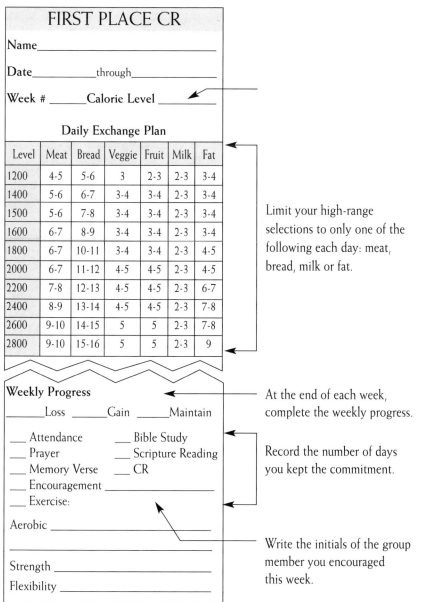

FIRST PLACE CR

Name_____

Date_____through_____

Week # _____Calorie Level _____

Daily Exchange Plan

Level	Meat	Bread	Veggie	Fruit	Milk	Fat
1200	4-5	5-6	3	2-3	2-3	3-4
1400	5-6	6-7	3-4	3-4	2-3	3-4
1500	5-6	7-8	3-4	3-4	2-3	3-4
1600	6-7	8-9	3-4	3-4	2-3	3-4
1800	6-7	10-11	3-4	3-4	2-3	4-5
2000	6-7	11-12	4-5	4-5	2-3	4-5
2200	7-8	12-13	4-5	4-5	2-3	6-7
2400	8-9	13-14	4-5	4-5	2-3	7-8
2600	9-10	14-15	5	5	2-3	7-8
2800	9-10	15-16	5	5	2-3	9

Weekly Progress

_____Loss _____Gain _____Maintain

___ Attendance   ___ Bible Study
___ Prayer   ___ Scripture Reading
___ Memory Verse   ___ CR
___ Encouragement _____
___ Exercise:

Aerobic _____

_____

Strength _____

Flexibility _____

Limit your high-range selections to only one of the following each day: meat, bread, milk or fat.

At the end of each week, complete the weekly progress.

Record the number of days you kept the commitment.

Write the initials of the group member you encouraged this week.

DAY 7: Date _____

Morning _____
_____
_____

Midday _____
_____
_____

Evening _____
_____
_____

Snacks _____
_____
_____

___ Meat _____   ☐ Prayer
___ Bread _____   ☐ Bible Study
___ Vegetable _____   ☐ Scripture Reading
___ Fruit _____   ☐ Memory Verse
___ Milk _____   ☐ Encouragement
___ Fat _____   ☐ Water_____

Exercise

Aerobic _____
_____

Strength _____

Flexibility _____

List the foods you have eaten. On this condensed CR it is not necessary to exchange each food choice. It will be the responsibility of each member that the tally marks you list below are accurate regarding each food choice. If you are unsure of an exchange, check the Live-It section of your copy of the *Member's Guide*.

List the daily food exchange choices to the left of the food groups.

Use tally marks for the actual food and water consumed.

Check off commitments completed. Use tally marks to record each 8-oz. serving of water.

List type and duration of exercise.

FIRST PLACE CR

Name _____

Date _____ through _____

Week # _____ Calorie Level _____

Daily Exchange Plan

Level	Meat	Bread	Veggie	Fruit	Milk	Fat
1200	4-5	5-6	3	2-3	2-3	3-4
1400	5-6	6-7	3-4	3-4	2-3	3-4
1500	5-6	7-8	3-4	3-4	2-3	3-4
1600	6-7	8-9	3-4	3-4	2-3	3-4
1800	6-7	10-11	3-4	3-4	2-3	4-5
2000	6-7	11-12	4-5	4-5	2-3	4-5
2200	7-8	12-13	4-5	4-5	2-3	6-7
2400	8-9	13-14	4-5	4-5	2-3	7-8
2600	9-10	14-15	5	5	2-3	7-8
2800	9-10	15-16	5	5	2-3	9

You may always choose the high range of vegetables and fruits. Limit your high range selections to only one of the following: meat, bread, milk or fat.

Weekly Progress

_____ Loss _____ Gain _____ Maintain

_____ Attendance _____ Bible Study
_____ Prayer _____ Scripture Reading
_____ Memory Verse _____ CR
_____ Encouragement:
_____ Exercise
Aerobic _____
Strength _____
Flexibility _____

DAY 5: Date _____

Morning _____

Midday _____

Evening _____

Snacks _____

_____ Meat
_____ Bread
_____ Vegetable
_____ Fruit
_____ Milk
_____ Fat

☐ Prayer
☐ Bible Study
☐ Scripture Reading
☐ Memory Verse
☐ Encouragement
Water _____

Exercise
Aerobic _____

Strength _____
Flexibility _____

DAY 6: Date _____

Morning _____

Midday _____

Evening _____

Snacks _____

_____ Meat
_____ Bread
_____ Vegetable
_____ Fruit
_____ Milk
_____ Fat

☐ Prayer
☐ Bible Study
☐ Scripture Reading
☐ Memory Verse
☐ Encouragement
Water _____

Exercise
Aerobic _____

Strength _____
Flexibility _____

DAY 7: Date _____

Morning _____

Midday _____

Evening _____

Snacks _____

_____ Meat
_____ Bread
_____ Vegetable
_____ Fruit
_____ Milk
_____ Fat

☐ Prayer
☐ Bible Study
☐ Scripture Reading
☐ Memory Verse
☐ Encouragement
Water _____

Exercise
Aerobic _____

Strength _____
Flexibility _____

DAY 1: Date _____

Morning _____

Midday _____

Evening _____

Snacks _____

___ Meat _____ ☐ Prayer
___ Bread _____ ☐ Bible Study
___ Vegetable _____ ☐ Scripture Reading
___ Fruit _____ ☐ Memory Verse
___ Milk _____ ☐ Encouragement
___ Fat _____
___ Water _____

Exercise
Aerobic _____
Strength _____
Flexibility _____

DAY 2: Date _____

Morning _____

Midday _____

Evening _____

Snacks _____

___ Meat _____ ☐ Prayer
___ Bread _____ ☐ Bible Study
___ Vegetable _____ ☐ Scripture Reading
___ Fruit _____ ☐ Memory Verse
___ Milk _____ ☐ Encouragement
___ Fat _____
___ Water _____

Exercise
Aerobic _____
Strength _____
Flexibility _____

DAY 3: Date _____

Morning _____

Midday _____

Evening _____

Snacks _____

___ Meat _____ ☐ Prayer
___ Bread _____ ☐ Bible Study
___ Vegetable _____ ☐ Scripture Reading
___ Fruit _____ ☐ Memory Verse
___ Milk _____ ☐ Encouragement
___ Fat _____
___ Water _____

Exercise
Aerobic _____
Strength _____
Flexibility _____

DAY 4: Date _____

Morning _____

Midday _____

Evening _____

Snacks _____

___ Meat _____ ☐ Prayer
___ Bread _____ ☐ Bible Study
___ Vegetable _____ ☐ Scripture Reading
___ Fruit _____ ☐ Memory Verse
___ Milk _____ ☐ Encouragement
___ Fat _____
___ Water _____

Exercise
Aerobic _____
Strength _____
Flexibility _____

Name _____

Date _____ through _____

Week # _____ Calorie Level _____

Daily Exchange Plan

Level	Meat	Bread	Veggie	Fruit	Milk	Fat
1200	4-5	5-6	3	2-3	2-3	3-4
1400	5-6	6-7	3-4	3-4	2-3	3-4
1500	5-6	7-8	3-4	3-4	2-3	3-4
1600	6-7	8-9	3-4	3-4	2-3	3-4
1800	6-7	10-11	3-4	3-4	2-3	4-5
2000	6-7	11-12	4-5	4-5	2-3	4-5
2200	7-8	12-13	4-5	4-5	2-3	6-7
2400	8-9	13-14	4-5	4-5	2-3	7-8
2600	9-10	14-15	5	5	2-3	7-8
2800	9-10	15-16	5	5	2-3	9

You may always choose the high range of vegetables and fruits. Limit your high range selections to only one of the following: meat, bread, milk or fat.

Weekly Progress

Loss _____ Gain _____ Maintain _____

_____ Attendance _____ Bible Study
_____ Prayer _____ Scripture Reading
_____ Memory Verse _____ CR
_____ Encouragement:
_____ Exercise
Aerobic _____
Strength _____
Flexibility _____

DAY 5: Date _____

Morning _____

Midday _____

Evening _____

Snacks _____

_____ Meat   ☐ Prayer
_____ Bread   ☐ Bible Study
_____ Vegetable ☐ Scripture Reading
_____ Fruit   ☐ Memory Verse
_____ Milk   ☐ Encouragement
_____ Fat   Water _____

Exercise
Aerobic _____

Strength _____
Flexibility _____

DAY 6: Date _____

Morning _____

Midday _____

Evening _____

Snacks _____

_____ Meat   ☐ Prayer
_____ Bread   ☐ Bible Study
_____ Vegetable ☐ Scripture Reading
_____ Fruit   ☐ Memory Verse
_____ Milk   ☐ Encouragement
_____ Fat   Water _____

Exercise
Aerobic _____

Strength _____
Flexibility _____

DAY 7: Date _____

Morning _____

Midday _____

Evening _____

Snacks _____

_____ Meat   ☐ Prayer
_____ Bread   ☐ Bible Study
_____ Vegetable ☐ Scripture Reading
_____ Fruit   ☐ Memory Verse
_____ Milk   ☐ Encouragement
_____ Fat   Water _____

Exercise
Aerobic _____

Strength _____
Flexibility _____

DAY 1: Date _____

Morning _____

Midday _____

Evening _____

Snacks _____

___ Meat ___   ☐ Prayer
___ Bread ___   ☐ Bible Study
___ Vegetable ___   ☐ Scripture Reading
___ Fruit ___   ☐ Memory Verse
___ Milk ___   ☐ Encouragement
___ Fat ___   ___ Water ___

Exercise
Aerobic _____
Strength _____
Flexibility _____

DAY 2: Date _____

Morning _____

Midday _____

Evening _____

Snacks _____

___ Meat ___   ☐ Prayer
___ Bread ___   ☐ Bible Study
___ Vegetable ___   ☐ Scripture Reading
___ Fruit ___   ☐ Memory Verse
___ Milk ___   ☐ Encouragement
___ Fat ___   ___ Water ___

Exercise
Aerobic _____
Strength _____
Flexibility _____

DAY 3: Date _____

Morning _____

Midday _____

Evening _____

Snacks _____

___ Meat ___   ☐ Prayer
___ Bread ___   ☐ Bible Study
___ Vegetable ___   ☐ Scripture Reading
___ Fruit ___   ☐ Memory Verse
___ Milk ___   ☐ Encouragement
___ Fat ___   ___ Water ___

Exercise
Aerobic _____
Strength _____
Flexibility _____

DAY 4: Date _____

Morning _____

Midday _____

Evening _____

Snacks _____

___ Meat ___   ☐ Prayer
___ Bread ___   ☐ Bible Study
___ Vegetable ___   ☐ Scripture Reading
___ Fruit ___   ☐ Memory Verse
___ Milk ___   ☐ Encouragement
___ Fat ___   ___ Water ___

Exercise
Aerobic _____
Strength _____
Flexibility _____

FIRST PLACE CR

Name _____

Date _____ through _____

Week # _____ Calorie Level _____

Daily Exchange Plan

Level	Meat	Bread	Veggie	Fruit	Milk	Fat
1200	4-5	5-6	3	2-3	2-3	3-4
1400	5-6	6-7	3-4	3-4	2-3	3-4
1500	5-6	7-8	3-4	3-4	2-3	3-4
1600	6-7	8-9	3-4	3-4	2-3	3-4
1800	6-7	10-11	3-4	3-4	2-3	4-5
2000	6-7	11-12	4-5	4-5	2-3	4-5
2200	7-8	12-13	4-5	4-5	2-3	6-7
2400	8-9	13-14	4-5	4-5	2-3	7-8
2600	9-10	14-15	5	5	2-3	7-8
2800	9-10	15-16	5	5	2-3	9

You may always choose the high range of vegetables and fruits. Limit your high range selections to only one of the following: meat, bread, milk or fat.

Weekly Progress

____ Loss   ____ Gain   ____ Maintain

____ Attendance   ____ Bible Study
____ Prayer   ____ Scripture Reading
____ Memory Verse   ____ CR
____ Encouragement: _____
____ Exercise
____ Aerobic
____ Strength
____ Flexibility

DAY 7: Date _____

Morning _____

Midday _____

Evening _____

Snacks _____

____ Meat   ☐ Prayer
____ Bread   ☐ Bible Study
____ Vegetable   ☐ Scripture Reading
____ Fruit   ☐ Memory Verse
____ Milk   ☐ Encouragement
____ Fat   ____ Water

Exercise
Aerobic _____
Strength _____
Flexibility _____

DAY 6: Date _____

Morning _____

Midday _____

Evening _____

Snacks _____

____ Meat   ☐ Prayer
____ Bread   ☐ Bible Study
____ Vegetable   ☐ Scripture Reading
____ Fruit   ☐ Memory Verse
____ Milk   ☐ Encouragement
____ Fat   ____ Water

Exercise
Aerobic _____
Strength _____
Flexibility _____

DAY 5: Date _____

Morning _____

Midday _____

Evening _____

Snacks _____

____ Meat   ☐ Prayer
____ Bread   ☐ Bible Study
____ Vegetable   ☐ Scripture Reading
____ Fruit   ☐ Memory Verse
____ Milk   ☐ Encouragement
____ Fat   ____ Water

Exercise
Aerobic _____
Strength _____
Flexibility _____

DAY 1: Date _____

Morning _____

Midday _____

Evening _____

Snacks _____

___ Meat	☐ Prayer
___ Bread	☐ Bible Study
___ Vegetable	☐ Scripture Reading
___ Fruit	☐ Memory Verse
___ Milk	☐ Encouragement
___ Fat	___ Water

Exercise
Aerobic _____
Strength _____
Flexibility _____

DAY 2: Date _____

Morning _____

Midday _____

Evening _____

Snacks _____

___ Meat	☐ Prayer
___ Bread	☐ Bible Study
___ Vegetable	☐ Scripture Reading
___ Fruit	☐ Memory Verse
___ Milk	☐ Encouragement
___ Fat	___ Water

Exercise
Aerobic _____
Strength _____
Flexibility _____

DAY 3: Date _____

Morning _____

Midday _____

Evening _____

Snacks _____

___ Meat	☐ Prayer
___ Bread	☐ Bible Study
___ Vegetable	☐ Scripture Reading
___ Fruit	☐ Memory Verse
___ Milk	☐ Encouragement
___ Fat	___ Water

Exercise
Aerobic _____
Strength _____
Flexibility _____

DAY 4: Date _____

Morning _____

Midday _____

Evening _____

Snacks _____

___ Meat	☐ Prayer
___ Bread	☐ Bible Study
___ Vegetable	☐ Scripture Reading
___ Fruit	☐ Memory Verse
___ Milk	☐ Encouragement
___ Fat	___ Water

Exercise
Aerobic _____
Strength _____
Flexibility _____

FIRST PLACE CR

Name _____

Date _____ through _____

Week # _____ Calorie Level _____

Daily Exchange Plan

Level	Meat	Bread	Veggie	Fruit	Milk	Fat
1200	4-5	5-6	3	2-3	2-3	3-4
1400	5-6	6-7	3-4	3-4	2-3	3-4
1500	5-6	7-8	3-4	3-4	2-3	3-4
1600	6-7	8-9	3-4	3-4	2-3	3-4
1800	6-7	10-11	3-4	3-4	2-3	4-5
2000	6-7	11-12	4-5	4-5	2-3	4-5
2200	7-8	12-13	4-5	4-5	2-3	6-7
2400	8-9	13-14	4-5	4-5	2-3	7-8
2600	9-10	14-15	5	5	2-3	7-8
2800	9-10	15-16	5	5	2-3	9

You may always choose the high range of vegetables and fruits. Limit your high range selections to only one of the following: meat, bread, milk or fat.

Weekly Progress

_____ Loss _____ Gain _____ Maintain

_____ Attendance _____ Bible Study
_____ Prayer _____ Scripture Reading
_____ Memory Verse _____ CR
_____ Encouragement:
_____ Exercise
_____ Aerobic
_____ Strength
_____ Flexibility

DAY 5: Date _____

Morning _____

_____

Midday _____

_____

Evening _____

_____

Snacks _____

_____

_____ Meat _____ ☐ Prayer
_____ Bread _____ ☐ Bible Study
_____ Vegetable _____ ☐ Scripture Reading
_____ Fruit _____ ☐ Memory Verse
_____ Milk _____ ☐ Encouragement
_____ Fat _____ Water _____

Exercise
Aerobic _____

Strength _____
Flexibility _____

DAY 6: Date _____

Morning _____

_____

Midday _____

_____

Evening _____

_____

Snacks _____

_____

_____ Meat _____ ☐ Prayer
_____ Bread _____ ☐ Bible Study
_____ Vegetable _____ ☐ Scripture Reading
_____ Fruit _____ ☐ Memory Verse
_____ Milk _____ ☐ Encouragement
_____ Fat _____ Water _____

Exercise
Aerobic _____

Strength _____
Flexibility _____

DAY 7: Date _____

Morning _____

_____

Midday _____

_____

Evening _____

_____

Snacks _____

_____

_____ Meat _____ ☐ Prayer
_____ Bread _____ ☐ Bible Study
_____ Vegetable _____ ☐ Scripture Reading
_____ Fruit _____ ☐ Memory Verse
_____ Milk _____ ☐ Encouragement
_____ Fat _____ Water _____

Exercise
Aerobic _____

Strength _____
Flexibility _____

DAY 1: Date _____

Morning _____

Midday _____

Evening _____

Snacks _____

___ Meat   ☐ Prayer
___ Bread   ☐ Bible Study
___ Vegetable ☐ Scripture Reading
___ Fruit   ☐ Memory Verse
___ Milk   ☐ Encouragement
___ Fat   ___ Water

Exercise
Aerobic _____
Strength _____
Flexibility _____

DAY 2: Date _____

Morning _____

Midday _____

Evening _____

Snacks _____

___ Meat   ☐ Prayer
___ Bread   ☐ Bible Study
___ Vegetable ☐ Scripture Reading
___ Fruit   ☐ Memory Verse
___ Milk   ☐ Encouragement
___ Fat   ___ Water

Exercise
Aerobic _____
Strength _____
Flexibility _____

DAY 3: Date _____

Morning _____

Midday _____

Evening _____

Snacks _____

___ Meat   ☐ Prayer
___ Bread   ☐ Bible Study
___ Vegetable ☐ Scripture Reading
___ Fruit   ☐ Memory Verse
___ Milk   ☐ Encouragement
___ Fat   ___ Water

Exercise
Aerobic _____
Strength _____
Flexibility _____

DAY 4: Date _____

Morning _____

Midday _____

Evening _____

Snacks _____

___ Meat   ☐ Prayer
___ Bread   ☐ Bible Study
___ Vegetable ☐ Scripture Reading
___ Fruit   ☐ Memory Verse
___ Milk   ☐ Encouragement
___ Fat   ___ Water

Exercise
Aerobic _____
Strength _____
Flexibility _____

FIRST PLACE CR

Name _____

Date _____ through _____

Week # _____ Calorie Level _____

Daily Exchange Plan

Level	Meat	Bread	Veggie	Fruit	Milk	Fat
1200	4-5	5-6	3	2-3	2-3	3-4
1400	5-6	6-7	3-4	3-4	2-3	3-4
1500	5-6	7-8	3-4	3-4	2-3	3-4
1600	6-7	8-9	3-4	3-4	2-3	3-4
1800	6-7	10-11	3-4	3-4	2-3	4-5
2000	6-7	11-12	4-5	4-5	2-3	4-5
2200	7-8	12-13	4-5	4-5	2-3	6-7
2400	8-9	13-14	4-5	4-5	2-3	7-8
2600	9-10	14-15	5	5	2-3	7-8
2800	9-10	15-16	5	5	2-3	9

You may always choose the high range of vegetables and fruits. Limit your high range selections to only one of the following: meat, bread, milk or fat.

Weekly Progress

_____ Loss _____ Gain _____ Maintain

_____ Attendance _____ Bible Study
_____ Prayer _____ Scripture Reading
_____ Memory Verse _____ CR
_____ Encouragement:
_____ Exercise
Aerobic

_____ Strength _____
_____ Flexibility _____

DAY 5: Date _____

Morning _____

Midday _____

Evening _____

Snacks _____

_____ Meat — ☐ Prayer
_____ Bread — ☐ Bible Study
_____ Vegetable — ☐ Scripture Reading
_____ Fruit — ☐ Memory Verse
_____ Milk — ☐ Encouragement
_____ Fat — Water _____

Exercise
Aerobic _____

Strength _____
Flexibility _____

DAY 6: Date _____

Morning _____

Midday _____

Evening _____

Snacks _____

_____ Meat — ☐ Prayer
_____ Bread — ☐ Bible Study
_____ Vegetable — ☐ Scripture Reading
_____ Fruit — ☐ Memory Verse
_____ Milk — ☐ Encouragement
_____ Fat — Water _____

Exercise
Aerobic _____

Strength _____
Flexibility _____

DAY 7: Date _____

Morning _____

Midday _____

Evening _____

Snacks _____

_____ Meat — ☐ Prayer
_____ Bread — ☐ Bible Study
_____ Vegetable — ☐ Scripture Reading
_____ Fruit — ☐ Memory Verse
_____ Milk — ☐ Encouragement
_____ Fat — Water _____

Exercise
Aerobic _____

Strength _____
Flexibility _____

DAY 1: Date _____

Morning _____

Midday _____

Evening _____

Snacks _____

☐ Prayer	Meat ___
☐ Bible Study	Bread ___
☐ Scripture Reading	Vegetable ___
☐ Memory Verse	Fruit ___
☐ Encouragement	Milk ___
	Fat ___ Water ___

Exercise
Aerobic _____
Strength _____
Flexibility _____

DAY 2: Date _____

Morning _____

Midday _____

Evening _____

Snacks _____

☐ Prayer	Meat ___
☐ Bible Study	Bread ___
☐ Scripture Reading	Vegetable ___
☐ Memory Verse	Fruit ___
☐ Encouragement	Milk ___
	Fat ___ Water ___

Exercise
Aerobic _____
Strength _____
Flexibility _____

DAY 3: Date _____

Morning _____

Midday _____

Evening _____

Snacks _____

☐ Prayer	Meat ___
☐ Bible Study	Bread ___
☐ Scripture Reading	Vegetable ___
☐ Memory Verse	Fruit ___
☐ Encouragement	Milk ___
	Fat ___ Water ___

Exercise
Aerobic _____
Strength _____
Flexibility _____

DAY 4: Date _____

Morning _____

Midday _____

Evening _____

Snacks _____

☐ Prayer	Meat ___
☐ Bible Study	Bread ___
☐ Scripture Reading	Vegetable ___
☐ Memory Verse	Fruit ___
☐ Encouragement	Milk ___
	Fat ___ Water ___

Exercise
Aerobic _____
Strength _____
Flexibility _____

FIRST PLACE CR

Name _____

Date _____ through _____

Week # _____ Calorie Level _____

Daily Exchange Plan

Level	Meat	Bread	Veggie	Fruit	Milk	Fat
1200	4-5	5-6	3	2-3	2-3	3-4
1400	5-6	6-7	3-4	3-4	2-3	3-4
1500	5-6	7-8	3-4	3-4	2-3	3-4
1600	6-7	8-9	3-4	3-4	2-3	3-4
1800	6-7	10-11	3-4	3-4	2-3	4-5
2000	6-7	11-12	4-5	4-5	2-3	4-5
2200	7-8	12-13	4-5	4-5	2-3	6-7
2400	8-9	13-14	4-5	4-5	2-3	7-8
2600	9-10	14-15	5	5	2-3	7-8
2800	9-10	15-16	5	5	2-3	9

You may always choose the high range of vegetables and fruits. Limit your high range selections to only one of the following: meat, bread, milk or fat.

Weekly Progress

_____ Loss _____ Gain _____ Maintain

_____ Attendance _____ Bible Study
_____ Prayer _____ Scripture Reading
_____ Memory Verse _____ CR
_____ Encouragement:
_____ Exercise
Aerobic _____

Strength _____
Flexibility _____

DAY 5: Date _____

Morning _____

Midday _____

Evening _____

Snacks _____

_____ Meat   ☐ Prayer
_____ Bread   ☐ Bible Study
_____ Vegetable   ☐ Scripture Reading
_____ Fruit   ☐ Memory Verse
_____ Milk   ☐ Encouragement
_____ Fat   _____ Water

Exercise
Aerobic _____

Strength _____
Flexibility _____

DAY 6: Date _____

Morning _____

Midday _____

Evening _____

Snacks _____

_____ Meat   ☐ Prayer
_____ Bread   ☐ Bible Study
_____ Vegetable   ☐ Scripture Reading
_____ Fruit   ☐ Memory Verse
_____ Milk   ☐ Encouragement
_____ Fat   _____ Water

Exercise
Aerobic _____

Strength _____
Flexibility _____

DAY 7: Date _____

Morning _____

Midday _____

Evening _____

Snacks _____

_____ Meat   ☐ Prayer
_____ Bread   ☐ Bible Study
_____ Vegetable   ☐ Scripture Reading
_____ Fruit   ☐ Memory Verse
_____ Milk   ☐ Encouragement
_____ Fat   _____ Water

Exercise
Aerobic _____

Strength _____
Flexibility _____

DAY 1: Date _____

Morning _____

Midday _____

Evening _____

Snacks _____

___ Meat   ☐ Prayer
___ Bread   ☐ Bible Study
___ Vegetable   ☐ Scripture Reading
___ Fruit   ☐ Memory Verse
___ Milk   ☐ Encouragement
___ Fat
___ Water _____

Exercise
Aerobic _____
Strength _____
Flexibility _____

DAY 2: Date _____

Morning _____

Midday _____

Evening _____

Snacks _____

___ Meat   ☐ Prayer
___ Bread   ☐ Bible Study
___ Vegetable   ☐ Scripture Reading
___ Fruit   ☐ Memory Verse
___ Milk   ☐ Encouragement
___ Fat
___ Water _____

Exercise
Aerobic _____
Strength _____
Flexibility _____

DAY 3: Date _____

Morning _____

Midday _____

Evening _____

Snacks _____

___ Meat   ☐ Prayer
___ Bread   ☐ Bible Study
___ Vegetable   ☐ Scripture Reading
___ Fruit   ☐ Memory Verse
___ Milk   ☐ Encouragement
___ Fat
___ Water _____

Exercise
Aerobic _____
Strength _____
Flexibility _____

DAY 4: Date _____

Morning _____

Midday _____

Evening _____

Snacks _____

___ Meat   ☐ Prayer
___ Bread   ☐ Bible Study
___ Vegetable   ☐ Scripture Reading
___ Fruit   ☐ Memory Verse
___ Milk   ☐ Encouragement
___ Fat
___ Water _____

Exercise
Aerobic _____
Strength _____
Flexibility _____

FIRST PLACE CR

Name _____

Date _____ through _____

Week # _____ Calorie Level _____

Daily Exchange Plan

Level	Meat	Bread	Veggie	Fruit	Milk	Fat
1200	4-5	5-6	3	2-3	2-3	3-4
1400	5-6	6-7	3-4	3-4	2-3	3-4
1500	5-6	7-8	3-4	3-4	2-3	3-4
1600	6-7	8-9	3-4	3-4	2-3	3-4
1800	6-7	10-11	3-4	3-4	2-3	4-5
2000	6-7	11-12	4-5	4-5	2-3	4-5
2200	7-8	12-13	4-5	4-5	2-3	6-7
2400	8-9	13-14	4-5	4-5	2-3	7-8
2600	9-10	14-15	5	5	2-3	7-8
2800	9-10	15-16	5	5	2-3	9

You may always choose the high range of vegetables and fruits. Limit your high range selections to only one of the following: meat, bread, milk or fat.

Weekly Progress

_____ Loss _____ Gain _____ Maintain

_____ Attendance _____ Bible Study
_____ Prayer _____ Scripture Reading
_____ Memory Verse _____ CR
_____ Encouragement:
_____ Exercise
Aerobic _____

Strength _____
Flexibility _____

DAY 5: Date _____

Morning _____

Midday _____

Evening _____

Snacks _____

_____ Meat   ☐ Prayer
_____ Bread   ☐ Bible Study
_____ Vegetable ☐ Scripture Reading
_____ Fruit   ☐ Memory Verse
_____ Milk   ☐ Encouragement
_____ Fat   _____ Water

Exercise
Aerobic _____

Strength _____
Flexibility _____

DAY 6: Date _____

Morning _____

Midday _____

Evening _____

Snacks _____

_____ Meat   ☐ Prayer
_____ Bread   ☐ Bible Study
_____ Vegetable ☐ Scripture Reading
_____ Fruit   ☐ Memory Verse
_____ Milk   ☐ Encouragement
_____ Fat   _____ Water

Exercise
Aerobic _____

Strength _____
Flexibility _____

DAY 7: Date _____

Morning _____

Midday _____

Evening _____

Snacks _____

_____ Meat   ☐ Prayer
_____ Bread   ☐ Bible Study
_____ Vegetable ☐ Scripture Reading
_____ Fruit   ☐ Memory Verse
_____ Milk   ☐ Encouragement
_____ Fat   _____ Water

Exercise
Aerobic _____

Strength _____
Flexibility _____

DAY 1: Date _____

Morning _____

Midday _____

Evening _____

Snacks _____

- ☐ Prayer
- ☐ Bible Study
- ☐ Scripture Reading
- ☐ Memory Verse
- ☐ Encouragement

____ Meat
____ Bread
____ Vegetable
____ Fruit
____ Milk
____ Fat
____ Water

Exercise
Aerobic _____
Strength _____
Flexibility _____

DAY 2: Date _____

Morning _____

Midday _____

Evening _____

Snacks _____

- ☐ Prayer
- ☐ Bible Study
- ☐ Scripture Reading
- ☐ Memory Verse
- ☐ Encouragement

____ Meat
____ Bread
____ Vegetable
____ Fruit
____ Milk
____ Fat
____ Water

Exercise
Aerobic _____
Strength _____
Flexibility _____

DAY 3: Date _____

Morning _____

Midday _____

Evening _____

Snacks _____

- ☐ Prayer
- ☐ Bible Study
- ☐ Scripture Reading
- ☐ Memory Verse
- ☐ Encouragement

____ Meat
____ Bread
____ Vegetable
____ Fruit
____ Milk
____ Fat
____ Water

Exercise
Aerobic _____
Strength _____
Flexibility _____

DAY 4: Date _____

Morning _____

Midday _____

Evening _____

Snacks _____

- ☐ Prayer
- ☐ Bible Study
- ☐ Scripture Reading
- ☐ Memory Verse
- ☐ Encouragement

____ Meat
____ Bread
____ Vegetable
____ Fruit
____ Milk
____ Fat
____ Water

Exercise
Aerobic _____
Strength _____
Flexibility _____

FIRST PLACE CR

Name _____

Date _____ through _____

Week # _____ Calorie Level _____

Daily Exchange Plan

Level	Meat	Bread	Veggie	Fruit	Milk	Fat
1200	4-5	5-6	3	2-3	2-3	3-4
1400	5-6	6-7	3-4	3-4	2-3	3-4
1500	5-6	7-8	3-4	3-4	2-3	3-4
1600	6-7	8-9	3-4	3-4	2-3	3-4
1800	6-7	10-11	3-4	3-4	2-3	4-5
2000	6-7	11-12	4-5	4-5	2-3	4-5
2200	7-8	12-13	4-5	4-5	2-3	6-7
2400	8-9	13-14	4-5	4-5	2-3	7-8
2600	9-10	14-15	5	5	2-3	7-8
2800	9-10	15-16	5	5	2-3	9

You may always choose the high range of vegetables and fruits. Limit your high range selections to only one of the following: meat, bread, milk or fat.

Weekly Progress

_____ Loss _____ Gain _____ Maintain

_____ Attendance

_____ Prayer _____ Bible Study

_____ Memory Verse _____ Scripture Reading

_____ Encouragement: _____ CR

_____ Exercise

_____ Aerobic

_____ Strength

_____ Flexibility

DAY 7: Date _____

Morning _____

Midday _____

Evening _____

Snacks _____

_____ Meat _____ Prayer
_____ Bread _____ Bible Study
_____ Vegetable _____ Scripture Reading
_____ Fruit _____ Memory Verse
_____ Milk _____ Encouragement
_____ Fat _____ Water

Exercise
Aerobic _____

Strength _____
Flexibility _____

DAY 6: Date _____

Morning _____

Midday _____

Evening _____

Snacks _____

_____ Meat _____ Prayer
_____ Bread _____ Bible Study
_____ Vegetable _____ Scripture Reading
_____ Fruit _____ Memory Verse
_____ Milk _____ Encouragement
_____ Fat _____ Water

Exercise
Aerobic _____

Strength _____
Flexibility _____

DAY 5: Date _____

Morning _____

Midday _____

Evening _____

Snacks _____

_____ Meat _____ Prayer
_____ Bread _____ Bible Study
_____ Vegetable _____ Scripture Reading
_____ Fruit _____ Memory Verse
_____ Milk _____ Encouragement
_____ Fat _____ Water

Exercise
Aerobic _____

Strength _____
Flexibility _____

DAY 1: Date _____

Morning _____

Midday _____

Evening _____

Snacks _____

___ Meat	☐ Prayer
___ Bread	☐ Bible Study
___ Vegetable	☐ Scripture Reading
___ Fruit	☐ Memory Verse
___ Milk	☐ Encouragement
___ Fat	

Exercise
Aerobic _____
Strength _____
Flexibility _____

Water ___

DAY 2: Date _____

Morning _____

Midday _____

Evening _____

Snacks _____

___ Meat	☐ Prayer
___ Bread	☐ Bible Study
___ Vegetable	☐ Scripture Reading
___ Fruit	☐ Memory Verse
___ Milk	☐ Encouragement
___ Fat	

Exercise
Aerobic _____
Strength _____
Flexibility _____

Water ___

DAY 3: Date _____

Morning _____

Midday _____

Evening _____

Snacks _____

___ Meat	☐ Prayer
___ Bread	☐ Bible Study
___ Vegetable	☐ Scripture Reading
___ Fruit	☐ Memory Verse
___ Milk	☐ Encouragement
___ Fat	

Exercise
Aerobic _____
Strength _____
Flexibility _____

Water ___

DAY 4: Date _____

Morning _____

Midday _____

Evening _____

Snacks _____

___ Meat	☐ Prayer
___ Bread	☐ Bible Study
___ Vegetable	☐ Scripture Reading
___ Fruit	☐ Memory Verse
___ Milk	☐ Encouragement
___ Fat	

Exercise
Aerobic _____
Strength _____
Flexibility _____

Water ___

FIRST PLACE CR

Name _____

Date _____ through _____

Week # _____ Calorie Level _____

Daily Exchange Plan

Level	Meat	Bread	Veggie	Fruit	Milk	Fat
1200	4-5	5-6	3	2-3	2-3	3-4
1400	5-6	6-7	3-4	3-4	2-3	3-4
1500	5-6	7-8	3-4	3-4	2-3	3-4
1600	6-7	8-9	3-4	3-4	2-3	3-4
1800	6-7	10-11	3-4	3-4	2-3	4-5
2000	6-7	11-12	4-5	4-5	2-3	4-5
2200	7-8	12-13	4-5	4-5	2-3	6-7
2400	8-9	13-14	4-5	4-5	2-3	7-8
2600	9-10	14-15	5	5	2-3	7-8
2800	9-10	15-16	5	5	2-3	9

You may always choose the high range of vegetables and fruits. Limit your high range selections to only one of the following: meat, bread, milk or fat.

Weekly Progress

_____ Loss _____ Gain _____ Maintain

_____ Attendance _____ Bible Study
_____ Prayer _____ Scripture Reading
_____ Memory Verse _____ CR
_____ Encouragement:
_____ Exercise
Aerobic _____

Strength _____
Flexibility _____

DAY 5: Date _____

Morning _____

Midday _____

Evening _____

Snacks _____

_____ Meat ☐ Prayer
_____ Bread ☐ Bible Study
_____ Vegetable ☐ Scripture Reading
_____ Fruit ☐ Memory Verse
_____ Milk ☐ Encouragement
_____ Fat _____ Water

Exercise
Aerobic _____

Strength _____
Flexibility _____

DAY 6: Date _____

Morning _____

Midday _____

Evening _____

Snacks _____

_____ Meat ☐ Prayer
_____ Bread ☐ Bible Study
_____ Vegetable ☐ Scripture Reading
_____ Fruit ☐ Memory Verse
_____ Milk ☐ Encouragement
_____ Fat _____ Water

Exercise
Aerobic _____

Strength _____
Flexibility _____

DAY 7: Date _____

Morning _____

Midday _____

Evening _____

Snacks _____

_____ Meat ☐ Prayer
_____ Bread ☐ Bible Study
_____ Vegetable ☐ Scripture Reading
_____ Fruit ☐ Memory Verse
_____ Milk ☐ Encouragement
_____ Fat _____ Water

Exercise
Aerobic _____

Strength _____
Flexibility _____

DAY 1: Date _____

Morning _____

Midday _____

Evening _____

Snacks _____

___ Meat ___ ☐ Prayer
___ Bread ___ ☐ Bible Study
___ Vegetable ___ ☐ Scripture Reading
___ Fruit ___ ☐ Memory Verse
___ Milk ___ ☐ Encouragement
___ Fat ___ ___ Water ___

Exercise
Aerobic _____
Strength _____
Flexibility _____

DAY 2: Date _____

Morning _____

Midday _____

Evening _____

Snacks _____

___ Meat ___ ☐ Prayer
___ Bread ___ ☐ Bible Study
___ Vegetable ___ ☐ Scripture Reading
___ Fruit ___ ☐ Memory Verse
___ Milk ___ ☐ Encouragement
___ Fat ___ ___ Water ___

Exercise
Aerobic _____
Strength _____
Flexibility _____

DAY 3: Date _____

Morning _____

Midday _____

Evening _____

Snacks _____

___ Meat ___ ☐ Prayer
___ Bread ___ ☐ Bible Study
___ Vegetable ___ ☐ Scripture Reading
___ Fruit ___ ☐ Memory Verse
___ Milk ___ ☐ Encouragement
___ Fat ___ ___ Water ___

Exercise
Aerobic _____
Strength _____
Flexibility _____

DAY 4: Date _____

Morning _____

Midday _____

Evening _____

Snacks _____

___ Meat ___ ☐ Prayer
___ Bread ___ ☐ Bible Study
___ Vegetable ___ ☐ Scripture Reading
___ Fruit ___ ☐ Memory Verse
___ Milk ___ ☐ Encouragement
___ Fat ___ ___ Water ___

Exercise
Aerobic _____
Strength _____
Flexibility _____

FIRST PLACE CR

Name _____

Date _____ through _____

Week # _____ Calorie Level _____

Daily Exchange Plan

Level	Meat	Bread	Veggie	Fruit	Milk	Fat
1200	4-5	5-6	3	2-3	2-3	3-4
1400	5-6	6-7	3-4	3-4	2-3	3-4
1500	5-6	7-8	3-4	3-4	2-3	3-4
1600	6-7	8-9	3-4	3-4	2-3	3-4
1800	6-7	10-11	3-4	3-4	2-3	4-5
2000	6-7	11-12	4-5	4-5	2-3	4-5
2200	7-8	12-13	4-5	4-5	2-3	6-7
2400	8-9	13-14	4-5	4-5	2-3	7-8
2600	9-10	14-15	5	5	2-3	7-8
2800	9-10	15-16	5	5	2-3	9

You may always choose the high range of vegetables and fruits. Limit your high range selections to only one of the following: meat, bread, milk or fat.

Weekly Progress

_____ Loss _____ Gain _____ Maintain

_____ Attendance _____ Bible Study
_____ Prayer _____ Scripture Reading
_____ Memory Verse _____ CR
_____ Encouragement:
_____ Exercise
Aerobic

Strength _____
Flexibility _____

DAY 5: Date _____

Morning _____

Midday _____

Evening _____

Snacks _____

_____ Meat ☐ Prayer
_____ Bread ☐ Bible Study
_____ Vegetable ☐ Scripture Reading
_____ Fruit ☐ Memory Verse
_____ Milk ☐ Encouragement
_____ Fat Water _____

Exercise
Aerobic _____

Strength _____
Flexibility _____

DAY 6: Date _____

Morning _____

Midday _____

Evening _____

Snacks _____

_____ Meat ☐ Prayer
_____ Bread ☐ Bible Study
_____ Vegetable ☐ Scripture Reading
_____ Fruit ☐ Memory Verse
_____ Milk ☐ Encouragement
_____ Fat Water _____

Exercise
Aerobic _____

Strength _____
Flexibility _____

DAY 7: Date _____

Morning _____

Midday _____

Evening _____

Snacks _____

_____ Meat ☐ Prayer
_____ Bread ☐ Bible Study
_____ Vegetable ☐ Scripture Reading
_____ Fruit ☐ Memory Verse
_____ Milk ☐ Encouragement
_____ Fat Water _____

Exercise
Aerobic _____

Strength _____
Flexibility _____

DAY 1: Date _____

Morning _____

Midday _____

Evening _____

Snacks _____

____ Meat ____   ☐ Prayer
____ Bread ____   ☐ Bible Study
____ Vegetable ____   ☐ Scripture Reading
____ Fruit ____   ☐ Memory Verse
____ Milk ____   ☐ Encouragement
____ Fat ____   Water ____

Exercise
Aerobic _____
Strength _____
Flexibility _____

DAY 2: Date _____

Morning _____

Midday _____

Evening _____

Snacks _____

____ Meat ____   ☐ Prayer
____ Bread ____   ☐ Bible Study
____ Vegetable ____   ☐ Scripture Reading
____ Fruit ____   ☐ Memory Verse
____ Milk ____   ☐ Encouragement
____ Fat ____   Water ____

Exercise
Aerobic _____
Strength _____
Flexibility _____

DAY 3: Date _____

Morning _____

Midday _____

Evening _____

Snacks _____

____ Meat ____   ☐ Prayer
____ Bread ____   ☐ Bible Study
____ Vegetable ____   ☐ Scripture Reading
____ Fruit ____   ☐ Memory Verse
____ Milk ____   ☐ Encouragement
____ Fat ____   Water ____

Exercise
Aerobic _____
Strength _____
Flexibility _____

DAY 4: Date _____

Morning _____

Midday _____

Evening _____

Snacks _____

____ Meat ____   ☐ Prayer
____ Bread ____   ☐ Bible Study
____ Vegetable ____   ☐ Scripture Reading
____ Fruit ____   ☐ Memory Verse
____ Milk ____   ☐ Encouragement
____ Fat ____   Water ____

Exercise
Aerobic _____
Strength _____
Flexibility _____

FIRST PLACE CR

Name _____

Date _____ through _____

Week # _____ Calorie Level _____

Daily Exchange Plan

Level	Meat	Bread	Veggie	Fruit	Milk	Fat
1200	4-5	5-6	3	3	2-3	3-4
1400	5-6	6-7	3-4	3-4	2-3	3-4
1500	5-6	7-8	3-4	3-4	2-3	3-4
1600	6-7	8-9	3-4	3-4	2-3	3-4
1800	6-7	10-11	3-4	3-4	2-3	4-5
2000	6-7	11-12	4-5	4-5	2-3	4-5
2200	7-8	12-13	4-5	4-5	2-3	6-7
2400	8-9	13-14	4-5	4-5	2-3	7-8
2600	9-10	14-15	5	5	2-3	7-8
2800	9-10	15-16	5	5	2-3	9

You may always choose the high range of vegetables and fruits. Limit your high range selections to only one of the following: meat, bread, milk or fat.

Weekly Progress

_____ Loss _____ Gain _____ Maintain

_____ Attendance _____ Bible Study
_____ Prayer _____ Scripture Reading
_____ Memory Verse _____ CR
_____ Encouragement:
_____ Exercise
_____ Aerobic

_____ Strength
_____ Flexibility

DAY 5: Date _____

Morning _____

Midday _____

Evening _____

Snacks _____

_____ Meat ☐ Prayer
_____ Bread ☐ Bible Study
_____ Vegetable ☐ Scripture Reading
_____ Fruit ☐ Memory Verse
_____ Milk ☐ Encouragement
_____ Fat _____ Water

Exercise
Aerobic _____

Strength _____
Flexibility _____

DAY 6: Date _____

Morning _____

Midday _____

Evening _____

Snacks _____

_____ Meat ☐ Prayer
_____ Bread ☐ Bible Study
_____ Vegetable ☐ Scripture Reading
_____ Fruit ☐ Memory Verse
_____ Milk ☐ Encouragement
_____ Fat _____ Water

Exercise
Aerobic _____

Strength _____
Flexibility _____

DAY 7: Date _____

Morning _____

Midday _____

Evening _____

Snacks _____

_____ Meat ☐ Prayer
_____ Bread ☐ Bible Study
_____ Vegetable ☐ Scripture Reading
_____ Fruit ☐ Memory Verse
_____ Milk ☐ Encouragement
_____ Fat _____ Water

Exercise
Aerobic _____

Strength _____
Flexibility _____

DAY 1: Date _____

Morning _____

Midday _____

Evening _____

Snacks _____

___ Meat ___	☐ Prayer
___ Bread ___	☐ Bible Study
___ Vegetable ___	☐ Scripture Reading
___ Fruit ___	☐ Memory Verse
___ Milk ___	☐ Encouragement
___ Fat ___	___ Water ___

Exercise
Aerobic _____

Strength _____

Flexibility _____

DAY 2: Date _____

Morning _____

Midday _____

Evening _____

Snacks _____

___ Meat ___	☐ Prayer
___ Bread ___	☐ Bible Study
___ Vegetable ___	☐ Scripture Reading
___ Fruit ___	☐ Memory Verse
___ Milk ___	☐ Encouragement
___ Fat ___	___ Water ___

Exercise
Aerobic _____

Strength _____

Flexibility _____

DAY 3: Date _____

Morning _____

Midday _____

Evening _____

Snacks _____

___ Meat ___	☐ Prayer
___ Bread ___	☐ Bible Study
___ Vegetable ___	☐ Scripture Reading
___ Fruit ___	☐ Memory Verse
___ Milk ___	☐ Encouragement
___ Fat ___	___ Water ___

Exercise
Aerobic _____

Strength _____

Flexibility _____

DAY 4: Date _____

Morning _____

Midday _____

Evening _____

Snacks _____

___ Meat ___	☐ Prayer
___ Bread ___	☐ Bible Study
___ Vegetable ___	☐ Scripture Reading
___ Fruit ___	☐ Memory Verse
___ Milk ___	☐ Encouragement
___ Fat ___	___ Water ___

Exercise
Aerobic _____

Strength _____

Flexibility _____

FIRST PLACE CR

Name _____

Date _____ through _____

Week # _____ Calorie Level _____

Daily Exchange Plan

Level	Meat	Bread	Veggie	Fruit	Milk	Fat
1200	4-5	5-6	3	2-3	2-3	3-4
1400	5-6	6-7	3-4	3-4	2-3	3-4
1500	5-6	7-8	3-4	3-4	2-3	3-4
1600	6-7	8-9	3-4	3-4	2-3	3-4
1800	6-7	10-11	3-4	3-4	2-3	4-5
2000	6-7	11-12	4-5	4-5	2-3	4-5
2200	7-8	12-13	4-5	4-5	2-3	6-7
2400	8-9	13-14	4-5	4-5	2-3	7-8
2600	9-10	14-15	5	5	2-3	7-8
2800	9-10	15-16	5	5	2-3	9

You may always choose the high range of vegetables and fruits. Limit your high range selections to only one of the following: meat, bread, milk or fat.

Weekly Progress

___ Loss   ___ Gain   ___ Maintain

___ Attendance   ___ Bible Study
___ Prayer   ___ Scripture Reading
___ Memory Verse   ___ CR
___ Encouragement:
___ Exercise
Aerobic

Strength _____
Flexibility _____

DAY 5: Date _____

Morning _____

Midday _____

Evening _____

Snacks _____

___ Meat   ☐ Prayer
___ Bread   ☐ Bible Study
___ Vegetable   ☐ Scripture Reading
___ Fruit   ☐ Memory Verse
___ Milk   ☐ Encouragement
___ Fat   ☐ Water

Exercise
Aerobic _____

Strength _____
Flexibility _____

DAY 6: Date _____

Morning _____

Midday _____

Evening _____

Snacks _____

___ Meat   ☐ Prayer
___ Bread   ☐ Bible Study
___ Vegetable   ☐ Scripture Reading
___ Fruit   ☐ Memory Verse
___ Milk   ☐ Encouragement
___ Fat   ☐ Water

Exercise
Aerobic _____

Strength _____
Flexibility _____

DAY 7: Date _____

Morning _____

Midday _____

Evening _____

Snacks _____

___ Meat   ☐ Prayer
___ Bread   ☐ Bible Study
___ Vegetable   ☐ Scripture Reading
___ Fruit   ☐ Memory Verse
___ Milk   ☐ Encouragement
___ Fat   ☐ Water

Exercise
Aerobic _____

Strength _____
Flexibility _____

DAY 1: Date _____

Morning _____

Midday _____

Evening _____

Snacks _____

___ Meat	☐ Prayer
___ Bread	☐ Bible Study
___ Vegetable	☐ Scripture Reading
___ Fruit	☐ Memory Verse
___ Milk	☐ Encouragement
___ Fat ___ Water	

Exercise
Aerobic _____

Strength _____
Flexibility _____

DAY 2: Date _____

Morning _____

Midday _____

Evening _____

Snacks _____

___ Meat	☐ Prayer
___ Bread	☐ Bible Study
___ Vegetable	☐ Scripture Reading
___ Fruit	☐ Memory Verse
___ Milk	☐ Encouragement
___ Fat ___ Water	

Exercise
Aerobic _____

Strength _____
Flexibility _____

DAY 3: Date _____

Morning _____

Midday _____

Evening _____

Snacks _____

___ Meat	☐ Prayer
___ Bread	☐ Bible Study
___ Vegetable	☐ Scripture Reading
___ Fruit	☐ Memory Verse
___ Milk	☐ Encouragement
___ Fat ___ Water	

Exercise
Aerobic _____

Strength _____
Flexibility _____

DAY 4: Date _____

Morning _____

Midday _____

Evening _____

Snacks _____

___ Meat	☐ Prayer
___ Bread	☐ Bible Study
___ Vegetable	☐ Scripture Reading
___ Fruit	☐ Memory Verse
___ Milk	☐ Encouragement
___ Fat ___ Water	

Exercise
Aerobic _____

Strength _____
Flexibility _____

FIRST PLACE CR

Name _____

Date _____ through _____

Week # _____ Calorie Level _____

Daily Exchange Plan

Level	Meat	Bread	Veggie	Fruit	Milk	Fat
1200	4-5	5-6	3	2-3	2-3	3-4
1400	5-6	6-7	3-4	3-4	2-3	3-4
1500	5-6	7-8	3-4	3-4	2-3	3-4
1600	6-7	8-9	3-4	3-4	2-3	3-4
1800	6-7	10-11	3-4	3-4	2-3	4-5
2000	6-7	11-12	4-5	4-5	2-3	4-5
2200	7-8	12-13	4-5	4-5	2-3	6-7
2400	8-9	13-14	4-5	4-5	2-3	7-8
2600	9-10	14-15	5	5	2-3	7-8
2800	9-10	15-16	5	5	2-3	9

You may always choose the high range of vegetables and fruits. Limit your high range selections to only one of the following: meat, bread, milk or fat.

Weekly Progress

____ Loss ____ Gain ____ Maintain

____ Attendance   ____ Bible Study
____ Prayer   ____ Scripture Reading
____ Memory Verse   ____ CR
____ Encouragement:
____ Exercise
____ Aerobic
____ Strength
____ Flexibility

DAY 5: Date _____

Morning _____

Midday _____

Evening _____

Snacks _____

____ Meat   ☐ Prayer
____ Bread   ☐ Bible Study
____ Vegetable   ☐ Scripture Reading
____ Fruit   ☐ Memory Verse
____ Milk   ☐ Encouragement
____ Fat   ____ Water

Exercise
Aerobic _____

Strength _____
Flexibility _____

DAY 6: Date _____

Morning _____

Midday _____

Evening _____

Snacks _____

____ Meat   ☐ Prayer
____ Bread   ☐ Bible Study
____ Vegetable   ☐ Scripture Reading
____ Fruit   ☐ Memory Verse
____ Milk   ☐ Encouragement
____ Fat   ____ Water

Exercise
Aerobic _____

Strength _____
Flexibility _____

DAY 7: Date _____

Morning _____

Midday _____

Evening _____

Snacks _____

____ Meat   ☐ Prayer
____ Bread   ☐ Bible Study
____ Vegetable   ☐ Scripture Reading
____ Fruit   ☐ Memory Verse
____ Milk   ☐ Encouragement
____ Fat   ____ Water

Exercise
Aerobic _____

Strength _____
Flexibility _____

DAY 1: Date _____

Morning _____

Midday _____

Evening _____

Snacks _____

____ Meat	☐ Prayer
____ Bread	☐ Bible Study
____ Vegetable	☐ Scripture Reading
____ Fruit	☐ Memory Verse
____ Milk	☐ Encouragement
____ Fat	____ Water

Exercise
Aerobic _____
Strength _____
Flexibility _____

DAY 2: Date _____

Morning _____

Midday _____

Evening _____

Snacks _____

____ Meat	☐ Prayer
____ Bread	☐ Bible Study
____ Vegetable	☐ Scripture Reading
____ Fruit	☐ Memory Verse
____ Milk	☐ Encouragement
____ Fat	____ Water

Exercise
Aerobic _____
Strength _____
Flexibility _____

DAY 3: Date _____

Morning _____

Midday _____

Evening _____

Snacks _____

____ Meat	☐ Prayer
____ Bread	☐ Bible Study
____ Vegetable	☐ Scripture Reading
____ Fruit	☐ Memory Verse
____ Milk	☐ Encouragement
____ Fat	____ Water

Exercise
Aerobic _____
Strength _____
Flexibility _____

DAY 4: Date _____

Morning _____

Midday _____

Evening _____

Snacks _____

____ Meat	☐ Prayer
____ Bread	☐ Bible Study
____ Vegetable	☐ Scripture Reading
____ Fruit	☐ Memory Verse
____ Milk	☐ Encouragement
____ Fat	____ Water

Exercise
Aerobic _____
Strength _____
Flexibility _____

CONTRIBUTORS

Jody Wilkinson, M.D., M.S., the writer of the Wellness Worksheets for this study, is a physician and exercise physiologist at the Cooper Institute in Dallas, Texas. He trained at the University of Texas Health Science Center in San Antonio, Texas, and Baylor University Medical Center in Dallas. Dr. Wilkinson conducts research on physical activity, nutrition and weight management and has worked with the American Heart Association to develop a health program. He believes strongly in using biblical teaching to motivate people to take care of their physical bodies and enjoy abundant living. Jody and his wife, Natalie, have been married 10 years and have two daughters, Jordan and Sarah, and twin sons, Joel and Cooper.

Scott Wilson, C.E.C., A.A.C., the author of the menu plans for this study, has been cooking professionally for 23 years. A certified executive chef with the American Culinary Federation, he currently works in the Greater Atlanta area as a personal chef and food consultant and is certified with the United States Personal Chef Association. Along with serving as the national food consultant for First Place, he is on the culinary program advisory board of the Art Institute in Atlanta. Scott has also authored two cookbooks, *Dining Under the Magnolia* and *Healthy Home Cooking*. He is also active in church work and enjoys spending time with his wife of 18 years, Jennifer, and their daughter, Katie.

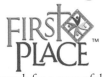
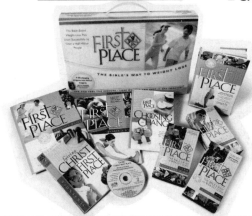
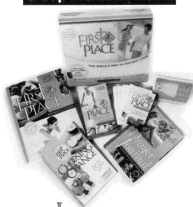

Bible Studies
to Help You Put Christ
First

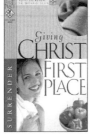

Giving Christ First Place
Bible Study
ISBN 08307.28643
Now Available

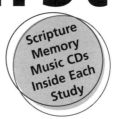

Scripture Memory Music CDs Inside Each Study

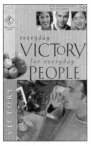

**Everyday Victory
for Everyday People**
Bible Study
ISBN 08307.28651

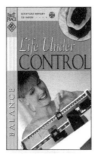

Life Under Control
Bible Study
ISBN 08307.29305

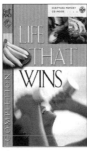

Life That Wins
Bible Study
ISBN 08307.29240

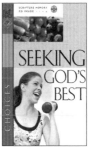

Seeking God's Best
Bible Study
ISBN 08307.29259

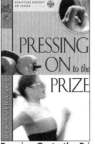

Pressing On to the Prize
Bible Study
ISBN 08307.29267

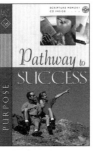

Pathway to Success
Bible Study
ISBN 08307.29275

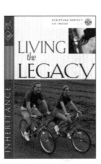

Living the Legacy
Bible Study
ISBN 08307.29283

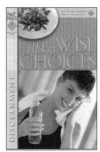

Making Wise Choices
Bible Study
ISBN 08307.30818

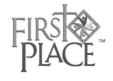

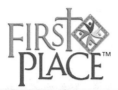

Available from your Gospel Light supplier

First Place Resource Order Form

TITLE	ISBN/SPCN	QTY	PRICE	ITEM TOTAL
First Place Group Starter Kit (S239 Value!)	08307.28708		149.99	
First Place Member's Kit (S101 Value!)	08307.28694		79.99	
First Place (included in Group Starter Kit)	08307.28635		18.99	
Choosing to Change (included in Member's and Group Starter Kits)	08307.28627		8.99	
Today Is the First Day	08307.30656		19.99	
Eating Healthy, Eating Right Meal Planner	08307.30222		18.99	
Health 4 Life	08307.30516		14.99	
Giving Christ First Place Bible Study w/Scripture Memory Music CD (included in Group Starter Kit)	08307.28643		19.99	
Everyday Victory for Everyday People Bible Study w/Scripture Memory Music CD	08307.28651		19.99	
Life That Wins Bible Study w/Scripture Memory Music CD	08307.29240		19.99	
Life Under Control Bible Study w/Scripture Memory Music CD	08307.29305		19.99	
Pressing On to the Prize Bible Study w/Scripture Memory Music CD	08307.29267		19.99	
Seeking God's Best Bible Study w/Scripture Memory Music CD	08307.29259		19.99	
Living the Legacy Bible Study w/Scripture Memory Music CD	08307.29283		19.99	
Pathway to Success Bible Study w/Scripture Memory Music CD	08307.29275		19.99	
Making Wise Choices Bible Study w/Scripture Memory Music CD	08307.30818		19.99	
Prayer Journal (included in Member's Kit)	08307.29003		9.99	
Motivational Audiocassettes (pkg. of 4) (included in Member's Kit)	607135.005988		29.99	
Commitment Records (pkg. of 13) (included in Member's Kit)	08307.29011		6.99	
Scripture Memory Verses: Walking in the Word (included in Member's Kit)	08307.28996		14.99	
Leader's Guide (included in Group Starter Kit)	08307.28678		19.99	
Food Exchange Plan Video (included in Group Starter Kit)	607135.006138		29.99	
Orientation Video (included in Group Starter Kit)	607135.005940		29.99	
Nine Commitments Video (included in Group Starter Kit)	607135.005957		39.99	
Giving Christ First Place Scripture Memory Music CD	607135.005902		9.99	
Giving Christ First Place Scripture Memory Music Cassette	607135.005919		6.99	
Everyday Victory for Everyday People Scripture Memory Music CD	607135.005926		9.99	
Everyday Victory for Everyday People Scripture Memory Music Cassette	607135.005933		6.99	
Life Under Control Scripture Memory Music CD	607135.006213		9.99	
Life Under Control Scripture Memory Music Cassette	607135.006206		6.99	
Life That Wins Scripture Memory Music CD	607135.006237		9.99	
Life That Wins Scripture Memory Music Cassette	607135.006220		6.99	
Seeking God's Best Scripture Memory Music CD	607135.006244		9.99	
Seeking God's Best Scripture Memory Music Cassette	607135.006251		6.99	
Pressing On to the Prize Scripture Memory Music CD	607135.006268		9.99	
Pressing On to the Prize Scripture Memory Music Cassette	607135.006275		6.99	
Pathway to Success Scripture Memory Music CD	607135.006282		9.99	
Pathway to Success Scripture Memory Music Cassette	607135.006299		6.99	
Living the Legacy Scripture Memory Music CD	607135.006305		9.99	
Living the Legacy Scripture Memory Music Cassette	607135.006312		6.99	
Making Wise Choices Scripture Memory Music CD	607135.007401		9.99	
Making Wise Choices Scripture Memory Music Cassette	607135.007418		6.99	

PRICES SUBJECT TO CHANGE. 11052

Total : $_____